KIDNEY DISEASE

DIET COOKBOOK FOR MEN

A Comprehensive Guide for the Newly Diagnosed With Kidney Friendly Meals For Controlled Sodium And Potassium, Regular Medical Monitoring And Follow-Up

Monalisa Blake

Copyright©2024 Monalisa Blake

All Rights Reserved. No part of this publication may be reproduced, distributed, or transmitted in any form or by any means, including photocopying, recording, or other electronic or mechanical methods without prior written permission of the publisher, except in the case of brief quotations embodied in critical reviews and certain other noncommercial uses permitted by copyright law.

TABLE OF CONTENT

INTRODUCTION 6
Importance of Diet in Managing Kidney Health 6
How This Cookbook Can Help 7
CHAPTER ONE 10
Understanding Kidney Disease 10
The Vital Role of Kidneys in the Body...10
Understanding the Nephrons: Basic Units of Kidney Function......................................10
Types of Kidney Disease And Causes:...10
Risk Factors for Kidney Disease 12
Diagnosis and Screening..12
Stages of Kidney Disease 12
Complications of Kidney Disease 13
Treatment Options..13
Lifestyle Modifications 13
Stages of Kidney Disease: From Early Detection to Advanced Stages 14
Common Symptoms and Complications of Kidney Disease 16
Importance of Early Diagnosis and Treatment in Kidney Disease 17
Chapter 2: Basics of Kidney-Friendly Nutrition 20
Nutritional Needs for Kidney Health 22
Understanding Sodium, Potassium, Phosphorus, and Fluid Intake in Kidney Health ..24
How to Read Food Labels for Kidney-Friendly Choices..26
Chapter 3: Meal Planning for Kidney Health 28
Portion Control and Serving Sizes 30
Chapter 4: Kidney-Friendly Cooking Techniques 32
Cooking Methods to Reduce Sodium and Phosphorus...33
Tips for Flavorful Seasoning without Adding Salt...34
Healthy Substitutions for High-Potassium Ingredients..36
Cooking Equipment and Tools for Kidney-Friendly Cooking 38
Chapter 5: Breakfast Recipes 40
Low-Sodium and Low-Phosphorus Breakfast Options..40
Protein-Rich Breakfast Ideas..44
Creative and Nutritious Smoothie Recipes 48

Chapter 6 .... *52*
Lunch and Dinner Recipes *52*

Kidney-Friendly Main Dishes with Lean Protein Sources 52
Delicious Side Dishes with Controlled Sodium and Potassium 2
Vegetarian and Vegan Options for Balanced Nutrition 3
One-Pot Meals for Easy Preparation and Cleanup 2

Chapter 7: Snacks and Appetizers *4*

Nutrient-Dense Snack Ideas for Kidney Health 4
Homemade Appetizers with Kidney-Friendly Ingredients 11
Portable Snacks for On-the-Go Convenience 13

Chapter 8: Desserts and Sweet Treats *16*

Low-Phosphorus Dessert Recipes for Indulgence without Compromise 19
Fruit-Based Desserts with Controlled Potassium 22
Tips for Enjoying Desserts in Moderation 25

Chapter 9: Beverages and Hydration *26*

Importance of Hydration for Kidney Function 27
Kidney-Friendly Beverage Options 28
Strategies for Monitoring Fluid Intake 29

Chapter 10: Managing Special Dietary Needs *32*

Diabetes and Kidney Disease: Dietary Considerations 34
Heart Health and Kidney Disease: Incorporating Heart-Healthy Eating 36
Gluten-Free and Dairy-Free Options for Dietary Restrictions 38
Strategies for Dining Out and Social Gatherings 40

Chapter 11: Lifestyle Tips for Kidney Health *42*

Exercise and Physical Activity Recommendations 43
Stress Management Techniques for Overall Wellness 44
Importance of Regular Medical Monitoring and Follow-Up Care 46

Encouragement and Support for Continued Success *48*
Conversion Charts for Nutritional Values *50*
Sample Grocery Lists *52*

INTRODUCTION

Managing kidney health, especially for those newly diagnosed with kidney disease, requires a multifaceted approach encompassing dietary modifications, lifestyle changes, regular medical monitoring, and follow-up care. This journey begins with understanding the vital role of kidneys in the body and the various types of kidney diseases, risk factors, and diagnostic procedures involved.

Throughout this process, individuals learn the importance of adopting a kidney-friendly diet, which emphasizes balanced nutrition, controlled intake of sodium, potassium, and phosphorus, and adequate hydration. They also discover the significance of lifestyle modifications, including regular exercise, stress management techniques, and strategies for maintaining a healthy weight and blood pressure.

Moreover, regular medical monitoring and follow-up care are paramount for early detection of kidney disease, assessment of kidney function, management of chronic conditions, prevention of complications, and optimization of treatment plans. These efforts are complemented by patient education, empowerment, and engagement in self-care practices to enhance overall kidney health and well-being.

By embracing these principles and working collaboratively with healthcare providers, individuals can navigate their journey with kidney disease more effectively, improve their quality of life, and empower themselves to take proactive steps towards better kidney health and overall wellness. Through continued education, support, and advocacy, we can strive to create a future where kidney disease is better understood, managed, and ultimately prevented, ensuring a brighter outlook for all individuals affected by this condition.

Importance of Diet in Managing Kidney Health

1. **Controlling Blood Pressure:** A diet low in sodium and high in potassium-rich foods such as fruits and vegetables can help lower blood pressure, reducing the risk of further kidney damage. High blood pressure is a common complication of kidney disease and can exacerbate existing kidney damage if left uncontrolled.

2. **Managing Fluid Balance:** Individuals with kidney disease may need to limit their fluid intake to prevent fluid retention and swelling (edema). Monitoring fluid intake, including beverages and foods with high water content, can help maintain fluid balance and prevent complications such as fluid overload and electrolyte imbalances.

3. **Reducing Protein Intake:** Protein metabolism produces waste products that the kidneys must filter out of the bloodstream. In individuals with kidney disease, reducing protein intake can help lessen the burden on the kidneys and slow the progression of

kidney damage. However, it's important to ensure that individuals still consume enough protein to meet their nutritional needs.

4. **Limiting Phosphorus and Potassium:** Impaired kidney function can lead to an accumulation of phosphorus and potassium in the bloodstream, potentially causing complications such as bone disorders and electrolyte imbalances. Restricting foods high in phosphorus and potassium, such as processed foods, dairy products, and certain fruits and vegetables, can help manage these levels and reduce the risk of complications.

5. **Monitoring Acid-Base Balance:** The kidneys play a crucial role in maintaining the body's acid-base balance by excreting excess acids or bases in the urine. In individuals with kidney disease, this balance may be disrupted, leading to metabolic acidosis. A diet low in acidic foods and high in alkaline foods, such as fruits and vegetables, can help support acid-base balance and reduce the risk of complications.

6. **Preventing Malnutrition:** Individuals with kidney disease are at increased risk of malnutrition due to dietary restrictions, reduced appetite, and metabolic changes. A well-balanced diet that provides adequate calories, protein, vitamins, and minerals is essential for preventing malnutrition and supporting overall health and well-being.

7. **Supporting Kidney Function:** Certain nutrients and dietary factors can either support or impair kidney function. For example, antioxidants found in fruits and vegetables can help protect the kidneys from oxidative stress and inflammation, while excessive consumption of certain nutrients, such as phosphorus and potassium, can strain kidney function.

How This Cookbook Can Help

Understanding the diagnosis of kidney disease can be overwhelming, but this cookbook serves as a valuable resource and companion on the journey toward better health. Here's how this cookbook can assist individuals newly diagnosed with kidney disease:

1. **Practical Guidance:** This cookbook offers practical guidance on how to navigate the dietary challenges associated with kidney disease. It provides clear explanations of dietary principles and practical tips for meal planning, grocery shopping, and dining out, making it easier for individuals to make informed choices about their nutrition.

2. **Kidney-Friendly Recipes**: The cookbook features a diverse selection of kidney-friendly recipes tailored to the nutritional needs of individuals with kidney disease. These recipes are designed to be delicious, satisfying, and easy to prepare, ensuring that individuals can enjoy flavorful meals without compromising their kidney health.

3. **Nutritional Information:** Each recipe is accompanied by detailed nutritional information, including sodium, potassium, and phosphorus content, allowing individuals to track their nutrient intake and make informed decisions about their dietary choices.

4. **Meal Plans:** The cookbook includes sample meal plans for different stages of kidney disease, providing individuals with a roadmap for planning balanced and nutritious meals that support kidney health. These meal plans take the guesswork out of meal planning and ensure that individuals are meeting their nutritional needs.

5. **Cooking Tips and Techniques:** In addition to recipes, the cookbook offers valuable cooking tips and techniques for preparing kidney-friendly meals. From reducing sodium and phosphorus to enhancing flavor without compromising on taste, these tips empower individuals to cook with confidence and creativity.

6. **Lifestyle Recommendations**: In addition to dietary guidance, the cookbook provides practical recommendations for lifestyle modifications that can support kidney health. From managing blood pressure to incorporating physical activity into daily routines, these recommendations help individuals take a holistic approach to managing their health.

7. **Empowerment and Support:** Above all, this cookbook aims to empower individuals with kidney disease to take control of their health and well-being. By providing practical tools, resources, and support, it instills confidence and optimism in individuals as they embark on their journey toward better kidney health.

CHAPTER ONE

Understanding Kidney Disease

Kidneys are remarkable organs with vital functions that are indispensable for maintaining overall health and well-being. This chapter provides a comprehensive overview of kidney health, covering the essential functions of the kidneys, various types of kidney diseases, associated risk factors, diagnostic methods, stages of kidney disease, complications, treatment options, and lifestyle modifications crucial for managing kidney health effectively.

The Vital Role of Kidneys in the Body

The kidneys play a crucial role in maintaining homeostasis within the body by performing several essential functions. These include filtration of waste products and toxins from the bloodstream, regulation of electrolyte levels, blood pressure, and fluid balance, as well as the production of hormones that regulate red blood cell production and blood pressure.

Understanding the Nephrons: Basic Units of Kidney Function

The nephron is the functional unit of the kidney responsible for filtering blood and producing urine. Each kidney contains millions of nephrons, comprising a renal corpuscle and renal tubule, which work together to filter and process waste products.

Types of Kidney Disease And Causes:

1. **Chronic Kidney Disease (CKD):** This progressive condition results in the gradual loss of kidney function over time.

   Causes:
   - Diabetes mellitus: Uncontrolled high blood sugar levels over time can damage the kidneys' filtering units (nephrons), leading to CKD.
   - Hypertension (high blood pressure): Persistent high blood pressure can strain the kidneys' blood vessels, causing damage and reducing kidney function.
   - Glomerulonephritis: Inflammation of the kidney's filtering units (glomeruli) can impair their function and contribute to CKD.
   - Polycystic kidney disease (PKD): Inherited disorder characterized by the growth of fluid-filled cysts in the kidneys, which can lead to kidney enlargement and loss of function.
   - Autoimmune diseases (e.g., lupus nephritis): Conditions where the immune system attacks the kidneys, causing inflammation and damage.
   - Recurrent kidney infections: Frequent or severe infections can scar the kidneys and impair their function over time.

2. **Acute Kidney Injury (AKI):** Characterized by a sudden and rapid decline in kidney function.

Causes:

- Severe dehydration: Inadequate fluid intake, excessive sweating, vomiting, or diarrhea can lead to dehydration and AKI.
- Medications: Certain medications, especially those that affect blood flow to the kidneys (e.g., NSAIDs, ACE inhibitors), can cause AKI.
- Infections: Severe infections such as sepsis can lead to AKI due to inflammation and decreased blood flow to the kidneys.
- Kidney obstruction: Blockages in the urinary tract, such as kidney stones or tumors, can prevent urine flow and cause AKI.
- Trauma: Physical injury to the kidneys, such as from accidents or surgeries, can result in AKI.
- Toxins: Exposure to certain toxins or chemicals, such as heavy metals or contrast dye used in imaging tests, can damage the kidneys and cause AKI.

3. **Polycystic Kidney Disease (PKD):** PKD is a hereditary condition characterized by the growth of fluid-filled cysts in the kidneys, leading to enlargement and impaired function.

Causes:

- Genetic mutations: PKD is an inherited disorder caused by mutations in genes responsible for kidney development and function.
- Autosomal dominant PKD (ADPKD): Most cases of PKD are inherited in an autosomal dominant pattern, meaning only one parent needs to pass on the mutated gene for the disease to occur.
- Autosomal recessive PKD (ARPKD): Less common and usually more severe form of PKD that is inherited in an autosomal recessive pattern, requiring both parents to carry the mutated gene.

4. **Glomerulonephritis:** This condition involves inflammation of the glomeruli, the tiny filters in the kidneys responsible for filtering waste and excess fluid from the blood.

Causes:

- Infections: Bacterial or viral infections, such as streptococcal infections (poststreptococcal glomerulonephritis) or viral hepatitis, can trigger glomerulonephritis.
- Autoimmune diseases: Conditions like lupus, IgA nephropathy, and Goodpasture syndrome involve the immune system attacking the glomeruli, leading to inflammation and damage.

- Genetic factors: Some forms of glomerulonephritis have a genetic predisposition, increasing the risk of developing the condition.
- Systemic diseases: Conditions like diabetes, hypertension, and vasculitis can affect the kidneys' blood vessels and contribute to glomerulonephritis.

5. **Other Kidney Conditions:**

- Kidney stones: Formed from crystals that accumulate in the kidneys, often due to dehydration, high calcium or uric acid levels, or certain medical conditions.
- Urinary tract infections (UTIs): Bacterial infections of the urinary tract, if left untreated, can spread to the kidneys and cause inflammation and damage.
- Renal artery stenosis: Narrowing of the arteries supplying blood to the kidneys, often due to atherosclerosis or fibromuscular dysplasia.
- Renal cell carcinoma: The most common type of kidney cancer, often developing from the cells lining the kidney tubules.

Risk Factors for Kidney Disease

Several factors increase the risk of developing kidney disease, including:

- **Diabetes Mellitus**: Uncontrolled diabetes can lead to diabetic nephropathy, a common cause of CKD.
- **Hypertension:** High blood pressure damages blood vessels in the kidneys, impairing their function over time.
- **Cardiovascular Disease:** Conditions such as heart disease and stroke can contribute to kidney damage.
- **Lifestyle Factors:** Smoking, obesity, poor diet, and sedentary behavior can all increase the risk of kidney disease.

Diagnosis and Screening

Early detection of kidney disease is crucial for initiating timely interventions to slow its progression. Common diagnostic tests include blood tests to assess kidney function (e.g., serum creatinine, estimated glomerular filtration rate), urinalysis to detect abnormalities in urine composition, and imaging studies (e.g., ultrasound, CT scan) to evaluate kidney structure and identify abnormalities.

Stages of Kidney Disease

Chronic kidney disease is categorized into five stages based on the severity of kidney damage and the level of kidney function, as determined by the estimated glomerular filtration rate (GFR). Each stage represents a progressively worsening condition, ranging from mild kidney damage

(Stage 1) to kidney failure (Stage 5), requiring renal replacement therapy such as dialysis or kidney transplantation.

Complications of Kidney Disease

Kidney disease can lead to various complications that affect other organ systems in the body, including:

- **Cardiovascular Complications:** Hypertension, heart disease, and stroke are common complications of kidney disease due to the interplay between kidney function and cardiovascular health.

- **Anemia:** Decreased production of erythropoietin, a hormone produced by the kidneys, can lead to anemia, characterized by low red blood cell counts and fatigue.

- **Bone Health and Mineral Metabolism:** Imbalances in calcium and phosphorus levels can lead to bone disorders such as osteoporosis and renal osteodystrophy.

- **Electrolyte Imbalance:** Impaired kidney function can disrupt the body's ability to regulate electrolyte levels, leading to abnormalities in sodium, potassium, and fluid balance.

Treatment Options

Treatment strategies for kidney disease aim to slow disease progression, manage symptoms, and prevent complications. These may include:

- **Medications:** ACE inhibitors, angiotensin II receptor blockers (ARBs), diuretics, phosphate binders, and erythropoiesis-stimulating agents are commonly prescribed to manage blood pressure, fluid balance, anemia, and mineral metabolism.

- **Dialysis Therapy:** Hemodialysis and peritoneal dialysis are renal replacement therapies that help remove waste products and excess fluid from the bloodstream in individuals with advanced kidney failure.

- **Kidney Transplantation:** Kidney transplantation offers a potential cure for kidney failure, providing a new kidney to replace the function of the diseased kidneys. Pre-transplant evaluation, surgery, and post-transplant care are integral parts of the transplantation process.

Lifestyle Modifications

In addition to medical interventions, lifestyle modifications are essential for managing kidney disease effectively. These may include:

- **Healthy Eating:** Following a balanced diet low in sodium, phosphorus, and potassium while emphasizing lean proteins, fruits, vegetables, and whole grains can help support kidney health.

- **Blood Pressure Management:** Adopting lifestyle changes such as reducing sodium intake, maintaining a healthy weight, and engaging in regular physical activity can help control hypertension and protect kidney function.

- **Smoking Cessation and Alcohol Moderation:** Quitting smoking and limiting alcohol consumption can reduce the risk of cardiovascular disease and kidney damage.

- **Physical Activity:** Regular exercise, as recommended by healthcare professionals, can improve cardiovascular health, manage weight, and enhance overall well-being.

Stages of Kidney Disease: From Early Detection to Advanced Stages

Chronic kidney disease (CKD) progresses through stages, each representing a different level of kidney function. Early detection and management are crucial for slowing the progression of CKD and preventing complications. The stages of kidney disease are typically determined based on the estimated glomerular filtration rate (eGFR), which measures how well the kidneys are filtering waste from the blood, as well as the presence of kidney damage.

1. **Stage 1:** Kidney Damage with Normal or High eGFR

    - In Stage 1 CKD, kidney damage is present, but kidney function is still normal or only slightly reduced.

    - Kidney damage may be detected through urine tests that show proteinuria (protein in the urine) or imaging studies that reveal structural abnormalities.

    - eGFR is equal to or greater than 90 mL/min/1.73 m².

    - Patients in this stage may not experience any symptoms, but they are at increased risk of developing kidney disease progression.

2. **Stage 2:** Mildly Reduced GFR

    - In Stage 2 CKD, kidney function is mildly reduced, indicating a slight decrease in kidney function.

    - eGFR is between 60 and 89 mL/min/1.73 m².

    - Kidney damage may progress, leading to increased proteinuria and further structural abnormalities.

    - Patients may still not experience noticeable symptoms, but they remain at risk of disease progression.

3. **Stage 3:** Moderately Reduced eGFR

    - Stage 3 CKD is divided into two sub-stages: a. Stage 3a: eGFR is between 45 and 59 mL/min/1.73 m². b. Stage 3b: eGFR is between 30 and 44 mL/min/1.73 m².

- Kidney function is moderately reduced, indicating significant impairment in kidney function.
- Patients may start experiencing symptoms such as fatigue, swelling (edema), and changes in urination patterns.
- Close monitoring and management are essential to slow disease progression and prevent complications.

4. **Stage 4:** Severely Reduced eGFR
    - In Stage 4 CKD, kidney function is severely reduced, indicating advanced kidney damage.
    - eGFR is between 15 and 29 mL/min/1.73 m².
    - Symptoms become more pronounced, including severe fatigue, fluid retention, shortness of breath, nausea, and decreased appetite.
    - Patients are at high risk of complications such as anemia, bone disorders, and cardiovascular disease.
    - Preparation for renal replacement therapy (dialysis or kidney transplantation) may be initiated in this stage.

5. **Stage 5:** Kidney Failure (End-Stage Renal Disease)
    - Stage 5 CKD, also known as end-stage renal disease (ESRD), is the most advanced stage of kidney disease.
    - eGFR is less than 15 mL/min/1.73 m² or the patient requires renal replacement therapy.
    - Kidney function is severely impaired or lost completely, resulting in the accumulation of waste products and toxins in the bloodstream.
    - Symptoms are severe and may include extreme fatigue, fluid overload, electrolyte imbalances, and uremia.
    - Renal replacement therapy (dialysis or kidney transplantation) is necessary to sustain life in this stage.

Common Symptoms and Complications of Kidney Disease

Kidney disease can manifest with a variety of symptoms and complications, ranging from mild to severe. Early detection and management of these symptoms are essential for preserving kidney function and preventing further complications. Here are some of the common symptoms and complications associated with kidney disease:

1. **Symptoms: a. Fatigue:** Feeling unusually tired or lacking energy, even after adequate rest. b. Swelling (Edema): Accumulation of fluid in the body, typically seen as swelling in the ankles, legs, hands, or face. c. Changes in Urination:

   - **Decreased urine output:** Producing less urine than usual or experiencing infrequent urination.
   - **Foamy or bubbly urine:** Presence of excess protein in the urine, known as proteinuria.
   - **Frequent urination:** Needing to urinate more often, especially at night (nocturia). d. Shortness of Breath: Difficulty breathing or feeling short of breath, particularly during physical exertion or while lying down. e. Nausea and Vomiting: Feeling nauseous or experiencing vomiting, often due to the accumulation of waste products and toxins in the bloodstream. f. Itching (Pruritus): Persistent itching of the skin, often without a visible rash, caused by the buildup of waste products in the blood. g. Muscle Cramps: Painful involuntary contractions of muscles, commonly occurring in the legs. h. Appetite Changes: Loss of appetite or changes in taste perception, leading to decreased food intake.

2. **Complications: a. Cardiovascular Complications:**

   - **Hypertension (High Blood Pressure):** Kidney disease can lead to elevated blood pressure, increasing the risk of heart disease, heart attack, and stroke.
   - **Heart Disease:** Chronic kidney disease is associated with an increased risk of cardiovascular events, such as coronary artery disease and heart failure. b. Anemia: Reduced production of red blood cells due to impaired kidney function, leading to symptoms such as fatigue, weakness, and pale skin. c. Bone Disorders:
   - **Osteoporosis:** Weakening of the bones, increasing the risk of fractures.
   - **Renal Osteodystrophy:** Imbalances in calcium and phosphorus levels, leading to bone pain, fractures, and deformities. d. Electrolyte Imbalances:
   - **Hyperkalemia:** Elevated potassium levels in the blood, which can cause irregular heartbeats and cardiac arrest.
   - **Hyponatremia:** Low sodium levels in the blood, leading to symptoms such as confusion, seizures, and coma. e. Fluid Overload: Accumulation of excess fluid in

the body, causing swelling, shortness of breath, and high blood pressure. f. Uremia: Buildup of waste products and toxins in the bloodstream, leading to symptoms such as fatigue, nausea, vomiting, and confusion. g. Endocrine Disorders: Kidney disease can disrupt hormone production, leading to complications such as insulin resistance, metabolic syndrome, and thyroid dysfunction.

Importance of Early Diagnosis and Treatment in Kidney Disease

Early diagnosis and treatment are paramount in the management of kidney disease, as they can significantly impact disease progression, complications, and overall outcomes. Here's why early intervention is crucial:

1. **Preservation of Kidney Function:**
   - Early detection allows healthcare providers to identify kidney disease in its initial stages when kidney function may still be preserved or only mildly impaired.
   - Prompt initiation of treatment can help slow or halt the progression of kidney disease, preserving kidney function and delaying the need for renal replacement therapy such as dialysis or transplantation.

2. **Prevention of Complications:**
   - Kidney disease is associated with various complications, including cardiovascular disease, anemia, bone disorders, electrolyte imbalances, and fluid overload.
   - Early diagnosis and treatment can help identify and manage these complications before they become severe, reducing the risk of long-term morbidity and mortality.

3. **Improved Quality of Life:**
   - Managing kidney disease early on can help alleviate symptoms such as fatigue, swelling, shortness of breath, and itching, improving overall quality of life for affected individuals.
   - Early intervention allows for the implementation of lifestyle modifications, dietary changes, and medications to help manage symptoms and optimize health outcomes.

4. **Delayed Progression to End-Stage Renal Disease (ESRD):**
   - ESRD represents the most advanced stage of kidney disease, requiring renal replacement therapy to sustain life.
   - Early diagnosis and treatment can help slow the progression of kidney disease, delaying or preventing the onset of ESRD and reducing the need for invasive and costly treatments such as dialysis or transplantation.

5. **Reduction of Healthcare Costs:**
    - Early detection and management of kidney disease can lead to cost savings by preventing complications, hospitalizations, and the need for intensive medical interventions.
    - Treating kidney disease in its early stages is generally less expensive and more cost-effective than managing complications associated with advanced kidney disease.

6. **Empowerment and Education:**
    - Early diagnosis provides an opportunity for individuals to become actively involved in their healthcare and make informed decisions about their treatment options.
    - Education about kidney disease, its causes, symptoms, and management strategies empowers individuals to take control of their health and adopt lifestyle changes that can slow disease progression and improve outcomes.

Chapter 2: Basics of Kidney-Friendly Nutrition

Kidney-friendly nutrition plays a crucial role in managing kidney disease and preserving kidney function. A well-planned diet can help reduce the burden on the kidneys, manage symptoms, prevent complications, and improve overall health outcomes. Here are the basics of kidney-friendly nutrition:

1. **Sodium Restriction:**

    - Limiting sodium intake is essential for managing fluid balance and blood pressure, which are critical in kidney disease.

    - Aim to consume less than 2,300 milligrams of sodium per day, or even less if advised by a healthcare provider.

    - Avoid high-sodium processed foods, canned soups, salty snacks, and cured meats.

    - Use herbs, spices, lemon juice, vinegar, and low-sodium seasoning blends to add flavor to meals without increasing sodium intake.

2. **Potassium Management:**

    - In advanced stages of kidney disease, potassium levels may become elevated, leading to complications such as irregular heartbeats.

    - Choose low-potassium fruits and vegetables, such as apples, berries, cabbage, green beans, and cauliflower.

    - Limit high-potassium foods like bananas, oranges, potatoes, tomatoes, and spinach.

    - Cooking methods such as boiling and leaching can help reduce potassium content in certain foods.

3. **Phosphorus Control:**

    - Elevated phosphorus levels in the blood can contribute to bone disorders and cardiovascular complications in kidney disease.

    - Avoid high-phosphorus foods such as dairy products, nuts, seeds, processed meats, and colas.

- Choose lower-phosphorus alternatives and limit portion sizes of high-phosphorus foods.
- Phosphate binders may be prescribed to help control phosphorus absorption from the diet.

4. **Protein Moderation:**
    - Reducing protein intake can help lessen the workload on the kidneys and slow the progression of kidney disease.
    - Focus on high-quality protein sources such as lean meats, poultry, fish, eggs, and plant-based proteins like beans and tofu.
    - Monitor portion sizes and limit protein intake to recommended levels based on individual needs and stage of kidney disease.
    - Consult with a registered dietitian to ensure adequate protein intake while managing kidney health.

5. **Fluid Management:**
    - Individuals with kidney disease may need to limit fluid intake to prevent fluid overload and swelling.
    - Monitor fluid intake and adhere to fluid restrictions recommended by a healthcare provider.
    - Choose thirst-quenching beverages such as water, herbal teas, and homemade lemonade while avoiding high-calorie and high-sugar drinks.
    - Limit consumption of foods with high water content, such as soups, fruits, and vegetables, if necessary.

6. **Phosphate Binder Use:**
    - Phosphate binders are medications prescribed to reduce phosphorus absorption from the diet and prevent complications in kidney disease.
    - Take phosphate binders as directed by a healthcare provider, typically with meals or snacks containing phosphorus-containing foods.
    - Follow dietary recommendations to minimize phosphorus intake and maximize the effectiveness of phosphate binders.

7. **Individualized Meal Planning:**
   - Work with a registered dietitian specializing in kidney disease to develop a personalized meal plan tailored to individual needs, preferences, and stage of kidney disease.
   - Monitor lab values regularly to assess kidney function and adjust dietary recommendations as needed.
   - Keep a food diary to track intake, symptoms, and adherence to dietary recommendations.

Nutritional Needs for Kidney Health

1. **Protein Intake:**
   - Protein is essential for muscle repair, immune function, and overall health. However, individuals with kidney disease may need to moderate their protein intake to reduce the workload on the kidneys.
   - Aim for high-quality protein sources such as lean meats, poultry, fish, eggs, and plant-based proteins like beans and tofu.
   - Limit consumption of high-protein foods and opt for portion control to meet individual protein needs while minimizing strain on the kidneys.
   - Work with a registered dietitian to determine appropriate protein intake based on stage of kidney disease, nutritional status, and other individual factors.

2. **Sodium Restriction:**
   - Sodium, found primarily in salt, plays a significant role in fluid balance and blood pressure regulation. Excess sodium intake can lead to fluid retention and hypertension, both of which can exacerbate kidney disease.
   - Limit sodium intake by avoiding processed and packaged foods, which often contain high levels of sodium.
   - Choose fresh, whole foods and use herbs, spices, lemon juice, and vinegar to flavor meals instead of salt.
   - Read food labels carefully and opt for low-sodium or sodium-free alternatives whenever possible.
   - Follow recommendations from healthcare providers or dietitians regarding daily sodium limits.

3. **Potassium Management:**
   - Potassium is an electrolyte that plays a vital role in muscle function, nerve transmission, and fluid balance. However, abnormal potassium levels can be dangerous for individuals with kidney disease, particularly in advanced stages.
   - Choose low-potassium fruits and vegetables such as apples, berries, cabbage, green beans, and cauliflower.
   - Limit high-potassium foods like bananas, oranges, potatoes, tomatoes, and spinach.
   - Cooking methods such as boiling and leaching can help reduce potassium content in certain foods.
   - Monitor potassium levels regularly and adjust dietary choices accordingly.

4. **Phosphorus Control:**
   - Phosphorus is a mineral that works in tandem with calcium to maintain bone health and other vital functions. However, elevated phosphorus levels can occur in kidney disease and contribute to bone disorders and cardiovascular complications.
   - Limit intake of high-phosphorus foods such as dairy products, nuts, seeds, processed meats, and colas.
   - Choose lower-phosphorus alternatives and limit portion sizes of high-phosphorus foods.
   - Take phosphate binders as prescribed by healthcare providers to help control phosphorus absorption from the diet.

5. **Fluid Management:**
   - Proper fluid balance is essential for kidney function and overall health. Individuals with kidney disease may need to monitor their fluid intake to prevent fluid overload and swelling.
   - Follow fluid restrictions recommended by healthcare providers or dietitians, taking into account individual needs and stage of kidney disease.
   - Choose thirst-quenching beverages such as water, herbal teas, and homemade lemonade while limiting high-calorie and high-sugar drinks.
   - Monitor symptoms of fluid overload, such as swelling, shortness of breath, and sudden weight gain, and adjust fluid intake accordingly.

6. **Individualized Meal Planning:**

- Work with a registered dietitian specializing in kidney disease to develop a personalized meal plan tailored to individual needs, preferences, and stage of kidney disease.

- Monitor lab values regularly to assess kidney function and adjust dietary recommendations as needed.

- Keep a food diary to track intake, symptoms, and adherence to dietary recommendations.

Understanding Sodium, Potassium, Phosphorus, and Fluid Intake in Kidney Health

Proper management of sodium, potassium, phosphorus, and fluid intake is crucial for individuals with kidney disease to maintain optimal health and slow the progression of kidney damage. Here's an overview of each nutrient and its role in kidney health:

1. **Sodium:**

    - Sodium is an electrolyte that plays a critical role in maintaining fluid balance, nerve function, and muscle contraction.

    - In individuals with kidney disease, excessive sodium intake can lead to fluid retention, swelling (edema), high blood pressure (hypertension), and cardiovascular complications.

    - **To manage sodium intake:**

        - Limit consumption of processed and packaged foods, which are often high in sodium.

        - Choose fresh, whole foods and use herbs, spices, lemon juice, and vinegar to flavor meals instead of salt.

        - Read food labels carefully and opt for low-sodium or sodium-free alternatives whenever possible.

        - Follow recommendations from healthcare providers or dietitians regarding daily sodium limits.

2. **Potassium:**

    - Potassium is another electrolyte that plays a crucial role in muscle function, nerve transmission, and maintaining proper heart rhythm.

    - In kidney disease, abnormal potassium levels can lead to dangerous heart rhythm disturbances (arrhythmias).

- **To manage potassium intake:**
  - Choose low-potassium fruits and vegetables such as apples, berries, cabbage, green beans, and cauliflower.
  - Limit consumption of high-potassium foods like bananas, oranges, potatoes, tomatoes, and spinach.
  - Use cooking methods such as boiling and leaching to reduce potassium content in certain foods.
  - Monitor potassium levels regularly and adjust dietary choices accordingly.

3. **Phosphorus:**
   - Phosphorus is a mineral that works in conjunction with calcium to maintain bone health, energy metabolism, and cellular function.
   - In kidney disease, elevated phosphorus levels can contribute to bone disorders (renal osteodystrophy) and cardiovascular complications.
   - **To control phosphorus intake:**
     - Limit consumption of high-phosphorus foods such as dairy products, nuts, seeds, processed meats, and colas.
     - Choose lower-phosphorus alternatives and limit portion sizes of high-phosphorus foods.
     - Take phosphate binders as prescribed by healthcare providers to help control phosphorus absorption from the diet.

4. **Fluid Intake:**
   - Proper fluid balance is essential for kidney function, blood pressure regulation, and overall health.
   - Individuals with kidney disease may need to monitor their fluid intake to prevent fluid overload, swelling, and electrolyte imbalances.
   - **To manage fluid intake:**
     - Follow fluid restrictions recommended by healthcare providers or dietitians, taking into account individual needs and stage of kidney disease.
     - Choose thirst-quenching beverages such as water, herbal teas, and homemade lemonade while limiting high-calorie and high-sugar drinks.
     - Monitor symptoms of fluid overload, such as swelling, shortness of breath, and sudden weight gain, and adjust fluid intake accordingly.

How to Read Food Labels for Kidney-Friendly Choices

1. **Pay Attention to Serving Size:**
    - The serving size listed on the food label indicates the amount of food typically consumed in one sitting.
    - Compare the serving size on the label to the portion you typically eat to ensure accurate nutrient intake.

2. **Check Total Sodium Content:**
    - Look for the sodium content per serving listed on the label.
    - Choose foods with lower sodium content, aiming for options with less than 140 milligrams per serving.

3. **Review Potassium Content:**
    - Check the potassium content per serving listed on the label.
    - Opt for foods with moderate potassium content, choosing options with less than 200 milligrams per serving, or as recommended based on individual needs and stage of kidney disease.

4. **Evaluate Phosphorus Content:**
    - Assess the phosphorus content per serving listed on the label.
    - Select foods with lower phosphorus content, aiming for options with less than 100 milligrams per serving, or as advised by healthcare providers or dietitians.

5. **Look for Phosphate Additives:**
    - Check the ingredient list for phosphate additives, which may appear as phosphoric acid, sodium phosphate, or calcium phosphate.
    - Limit consumption of foods with phosphate additives, as they can contribute to elevated phosphorus levels in the blood.

6. **Consider Protein Content:**
    - Evaluate the protein content per serving listed on the label.
    - Choose foods with moderate protein content, especially if following a renal diet with protein restrictions.
    - Opt for high-quality protein sources such as lean meats, poultry, fish, eggs, and plant-based proteins like beans and tofu.

7. **Monitor Sugar and Fat Content:**

    - Pay attention to the sugar and fat content per serving listed on the label.
    - Limit consumption of foods high in added sugars and unhealthy fats, which can contribute to weight gain, diabetes, and cardiovascular disease, all of which can impact kidney health.

8. **Check for Allergens and Additives:**

    - Scan the ingredient list for potential allergens or additives that may be harmful or trigger adverse reactions.
    - Avoid foods containing ingredients that may exacerbate kidney disease symptoms or interact with medications.

9. **Seek "Kidney-Friendly" Labeling:**

    - Look for products labeled as "kidney-friendly" or "renal-friendly," which may indicate that the product is formulated with lower sodium, potassium, and phosphorus content.
    - Be cautious and still verify the nutrient content on the food label to ensure it aligns with individual dietary needs and restrictions.

Chapter 3: Meal Planning for Kidney Health

Meal planning is essential for individuals with kidney disease to ensure they are consuming a balanced diet that supports kidney health while managing nutrient intake and avoiding foods that may exacerbate their condition. Here's a guide to meal planning for kidney health:

1. **Assess Nutritional Needs:**

    - Work with a registered dietitian specializing in kidney disease to determine individual nutritional needs based on stage of kidney disease, lab results, medical history, and lifestyle factors.

    - Consider dietary restrictions such as sodium, potassium, phosphorus, and protein intake limits when planning meals.

2. **Create Balanced Meals:**

    - Aim for balanced meals that include a variety of food groups: lean protein, carbohydrates, healthy fats, fruits, and vegetables.

    - Incorporate high-quality protein sources such as lean meats, poultry, fish, eggs, dairy, and plant-based proteins like beans and tofu.

    - Choose complex carbohydrates such as whole grains, fruits, and vegetables, which provide fiber and essential nutrients.

3. **Monitor Portion Sizes:**

    - Pay attention to portion sizes to ensure moderation and prevent overeating, especially of foods high in sodium, potassium, and phosphorus.

    - Use measuring cups, scales, or visual cues to estimate portion sizes and avoid excessive intake of protein, grains, and high-potassium fruits and vegetables.

4. **Control Sodium Intake:**

    - Limit the use of salt and high-sodium seasonings in meal preparation.

    - Use herbs, spices, lemon juice, vinegar, and low-sodium seasoning blends to add flavor to meals without increasing sodium content.

    - Choose low-sodium or no-salt-added canned goods, broths, and condiments, and rinse canned foods under water before use to reduce sodium content.

5. **Manage Potassium and Phosphorus:**
   - Choose low-potassium fruits and vegetables, such as apples, berries, cabbage, green beans, and cauliflower, and limit high-potassium options like bananas, oranges, potatoes, tomatoes, and spinach.
   - Opt for low-phosphorus protein sources and limit consumption of high-phosphorus foods such as dairy products, nuts, seeds, processed meats, and colas.
   - Monitor phosphorus additives in processed foods and choose phosphate binder medications as prescribed by healthcare providers to control phosphorus absorption from the diet.

6. **Include Kidney-Friendly Snacks:**
   - Plan nutritious snacks that align with dietary restrictions, such as fresh fruit, raw vegetables with hummus, unsalted nuts, low-fat yogurt, air-popped popcorn, or whole grain crackers with cheese.
   - Portion snacks appropriately and avoid high-sodium, high-potassium, and high-phosphorus options.

7. Stay Hydrated:
   - Drink adequate fluids throughout the day to maintain hydration and support kidney function.
   - Choose water, herbal tea, and homemade lemonade as primary beverage options, and limit consumption of sugary drinks, caffeinated beverages, and alcohol.

8. **Be Flexible and Enjoy Variety:**
   - Experiment with different recipes, cooking methods, and flavor combinations to keep meals interesting and enjoyable.
   - Don't be afraid to modify recipes to meet individual dietary needs and preferences, substituting ingredients and adjusting portion sizes as needed.

9. **Plan Ahead and Batch Cook:**
   - Plan meals for the week ahead of time and create a grocery list based on planned recipes and nutritional needs.
   - Consider batch cooking and meal prep to save time and ensure healthy options are readily available throughout the week.
   - Store prepared meals and snacks in portioned containers for easy grab-and-go convenience.

Portion Control and Serving Sizes

1. **Use Visual Cues:**

   - Visualize portion sizes using common objects or your hand to estimate appropriate Servings:

     - A serving of meat or poultry is about the size of a deck of cards or the palm of your hand.

     - A serving of fish is about the size of a checkbook.

     - A serving of grains or starches is about the size of a baseball or your clenched fist.

     - A serving of fruits or vegetables is about the size of a tennis ball or your cupped hand.

     - A serving of cheese is about the size of four stacked dice or your thumb.

2. **Read Food Labels:**

   - Check food labels for information on serving sizes and nutrient content per serving.

   - Pay attention to the number of servings per package and adjust portion sizes accordingly to avoid overconsumption.

3. **Measure and Weigh Foods:**

   - Use measuring cups, spoons, and a kitchen scale to accurately portion foods and ingredients.

   - Measure out serving sizes of grains, cereals, pasta, and other dry goods to ensure proper portion control.

   - Weigh meat, poultry, fish, and other protein sources to meet individual dietary needs and recommendations.

4. **Be Mindful of Portion Distortion:**

   - Be aware of portion distortion, where oversized servings become the norm and contribute to overeating.

   - Resist the urge to supersize meals or indulge in oversized portions at restaurants and fast-food establishments.

5. **Split Larger Portions:**

   - Share larger meals with a dining companion or ask for a to-go container to divide portions and save leftovers for another meal.

- When dining out, consider splitting entrees or ordering appetizers or side dishes instead of full-sized meals.

6. **Fill Half Your Plate with Fruits and Vegetables:**
   - Aim to fill half your plate with colorful fruits and vegetables at each meal to increase nutrient intake and promote satiety.
   - Choose a variety of fresh, frozen, or canned fruits and vegetables to add flavor, texture, and nutritional value to your meals.

7. **Practice Mindful Eating:**
   - Pay attention to hunger and fullness cues, and eat slowly to savor flavors and enjoy your meals.
   - Pause between bites, and check in with your body to determine if you're satisfied or still hungry before reaching for seconds.

8. **Use Smaller Plates and Bowls:**
   - Opt for smaller plates, bowls, and utensils to visually trick your brain into thinking you're eating larger portions.
   - Avoid serving meals family-style from large serving dishes, as it can lead to overeating.

9. **Plan Ahead:**
   - Plan meals and snacks in advance, and portion out foods into individual servings or containers for easy grab-and-go convenience.
   - Prepare homemade meals using fresh, whole ingredients to control portion sizes and nutrient content.

Chapter 4: Kidney-Friendly Cooking Techniques

1. **Steaming:** Steaming is a gentle cooking method that helps preserve the natural flavors, textures, and nutrients of foods without the need for added fats or oils. Steam vegetables, fish, poultry, or grains using a steamer basket or microwave steaming bags for a simple and healthy cooking option.

2. **Boiling:** Boiling is a versatile cooking technique that can be used to cook pasta, grains, legumes, and vegetables. To minimize nutrient loss, use minimal water and avoid overcooking. Save the cooking liquid (broth) for soups or sauces to retain nutrients and flavor.

3. **Poaching:** Poaching involves cooking food gently in liquid at a low temperature, preserving moisture and tenderness. Poach fish, chicken, or eggs in water, broth, or a flavorful liquid like lemon juice or wine for a delicate and kidney-friendly preparation.

4. **Baking and Roasting:** Baking and roasting are dry heat cooking methods that can be used to cook meats, poultry, fish, vegetables, and fruits. Use minimal oil or fat and seasonings to enhance flavor while reducing sodium intake. Roasting vegetables at high heat caramelizes natural sugars, intensifying their flavors without the need for added salt or sugar.

5. **Grilling and Broiling:** Grilling and broiling are quick and convenient cooking techniques that impart smoky, charred flavors to foods. Grill or broil lean meats, poultry, fish, and vegetables without added marinades or sauces to minimize sodium and phosphorus content. Use herbs, spices, and citrus juices for flavor instead.

6. **Stir-Frying:** Stir-frying involves cooking small pieces of food quickly in a hot pan with minimal oil. Use heart-healthy oils like olive, avocado, or canola oil and incorporate a variety of colorful vegetables, lean proteins, and whole grains for a nutrient-rich meal. Avoid high-sodium sauces and seasonings, opting for low-sodium alternatives or homemade marinades.

7. **Slow Cooking:** Slow cooking is a convenient method for tenderizing tough cuts of meat, beans, and legumes while infusing flavors over an extended period. Use a slow cooker or crockpot to prepare kidney-friendly stews, soups, chili, and casseroles with lean proteins, whole grains, and plenty of vegetables. Choose low-sodium broths and seasonings to control sodium intake.

8. **Blanching:** Blanching involves briefly boiling vegetables before shocking them in ice water to halt the cooking process. Blanching helps preserve color, texture, and nutrients while reducing potassium content in certain vegetables like potatoes and tomatoes.

9. **Microwaving:** Microwaving is a quick and convenient cooking method that requires minimal added fats or oils. Use microwave-safe containers to steam vegetables, cook grains, and reheat leftovers for a kidney-friendly meal in minutes.

Cooking Methods to Reduce Sodium and Phosphorus

1. **Rinsing and Soaking:**
   - Rinse canned beans, vegetables, and other canned foods under running water to remove excess sodium.
   - Soak high-phosphorus foods like beans, lentils, and grains in water overnight before cooking to reduce phosphorus content.

2. **Boiling and Draining:**
   - Boil high-sodium foods like canned vegetables or processed meats in water for a few minutes, then drain and rinse under cold water to reduce sodium content.
   - Boil potatoes, which are high in potassium, to reduce potassium content. Discard the cooking water to remove some of the potassium.

3. **Using Fresh Ingredients:**
   - Opt for fresh fruits, vegetables, and meats instead of canned or processed options, which often contain added sodium and phosphorus.
   - Choose fresh herbs, spices, and citrus juices to season foods instead of high-sodium sauces, marinades, or seasoning blends.

4. **Choosing Low-Sodium Ingredients:**
   - Select low-sodium or no-salt-added versions of canned goods, broths, condiments, and prepared foods whenever possible.
   - Look for low-phosphorus alternatives to high-phosphorus foods, such as low-phosphorus dairy products or phosphate-free baking powder.

5. **Herb and Spice Blends:**
   - Create homemade herb and spice blends using salt-free seasonings to flavor foods without adding sodium.

- Experiment with combinations of garlic powder, onion powder, black pepper, paprika, cumin, turmeric, and other herbs and spices to enhance taste.

6. **Limiting Salt and Salt Substitutes:**
   - Use salt sparingly in cooking and at the table, and gradually reduce salt amounts over time to adjust to lower sodium levels.
   - Avoid using salt substitutes containing potassium chloride if you need to limit potassium intake, and consult with your healthcare provider or dietitian for suitable alternatives.

7. **Grilling and Roasting:**
   - Grill or roast meats, poultry, fish, and vegetables with minimal seasoning to enhance natural flavors without relying on added salt or high-phosphorus ingredients.
   - Use non-stick cooking spray or a small amount of heart-healthy oil to prevent sticking without adding excess fat or sodium.

8. **Homemade Broths and Stocks:**
   - Prepare homemade broths and stocks using fresh vegetables, herbs, and lean cuts of meat to control sodium content.
   - Skim off fat and foam during cooking and strain the broth before using it in recipes to remove excess sodium and phosphorus.

9. **Portion Control:**
   - Monitor portion sizes to avoid overconsumption of high-sodium or high-phosphorus foods, especially processed foods, cured meats, cheese, and high-phosphorus additives.

Tips for Flavorful Seasoning without Adding Salt

1. **Fresh Herbs:** Fresh herbs add vibrant flavor and aroma to dishes without the need for salt. Experiment with basil, cilantro, parsley, dill, mint, rosemary, thyme, sage, and chives to enhance the taste of your meals. Add fresh herbs at the end of cooking or as a garnish to preserve their delicate flavors.

2. **Dried Herbs and Spices:** Dried herbs and spices are pantry staples that can elevate the flavor of your dishes without adding salt. Keep a variety of dried herbs and spices on hand, such as oregano, basil, garlic powder, onion powder, paprika, cumin, cinnamon, ginger, and turmeric. Use them generously to season meats, poultry, seafood, vegetables, soups, stews, and sauces.

3. **Citrus Zest and Juice:** Citrus zest and juice are excellent alternatives to salt for adding brightness and acidity to dishes. Use a microplane grater to zest lemons, limes, and oranges, and sprinkle the zest over salads, grilled meats, fish, and vegetables. Squeeze fresh citrus juice over cooked dishes or incorporate it into marinades, dressings, and sauces for a tangy flavor boost.

4. **Vinegars:** Vinegars, such as balsamic vinegar, apple cider vinegar, red wine vinegar, and rice vinegar, can add acidity and depth to your cooking without the need for salt. Use vinegar to make flavorful salad dressings, marinades, pickles, and sauces, or drizzle it over roasted vegetables, grilled meats, and seafood.

5. **Aromatics:** Aromatics like onions, garlic, shallots, and leeks are essential flavor builders in cooking. Sauté aromatics in a small amount of olive oil or vegetable broth until soft and fragrant, then use them as a base for soups, stews, sauces, and stir-fries. Their natural sweetness and complexity will enhance the overall flavor of your dishes.

6. **Homemade Spice Blends:** Create your own salt-free spice blends to season meats, poultry, fish, vegetables, and grains. Mix together your favorite dried herbs and spices, such as Italian seasoning, Cajun seasoning, curry powder, or chili powder, and store them in airtight containers for easy use.

7. **Umami-Boosting Ingredients:** Incorporate umami-rich ingredients like mushrooms, tomatoes, soy sauce (choose low-sodium options), miso paste, nutritional yeast, and Worcestershire sauce into your cooking to enhance flavor without salt. These ingredients add depth and savory notes to dishes, making them more satisfying and delicious.

8. **Toasted Nuts and Seeds:** Toasted nuts and seeds add crunch, texture, and nutty flavor to salads, grain dishes, and vegetable sautés. Experiment with toasted almonds, walnuts, pecans, pumpkin seeds, sesame seeds, or sunflower seeds to enhance the taste and nutritional value of your meals.

9. **Herbal Infused Oils:** Infuse olive oil or other heart-healthy oils with fresh herbs, garlic, chili flakes, or citrus zest to create flavorful finishing oils for drizzling over cooked dishes. Use herb-infused oils as a finishing touch to soups, salads, roasted vegetables, pasta dishes, and grilled meats.

10. **Nutritional Yeast:** Nutritional yeast is a versatile ingredient that adds a cheesy, savory flavor to dishes without the need for salt. Sprinkle nutritional yeast over popcorn, pasta, roasted vegetables, or homemade kale chips for a delicious umami boost.

Healthy Substitutions for High-Potassium Ingredients

1. **Potatoes:**
   - Substitute white potatoes with lower-potassium alternatives such as sweet potatoes or yams.
   - Try using cauliflower or turnips as a lower-potassium substitute for mashed potatoes.

2. **Tomatoes:**
   - Replace fresh tomatoes with low-potassium vegetables like bell peppers, cucumbers, or zucchini in salads and sandwiches.
   - Use roasted red bell peppers or sun-dried tomatoes (in moderation) for a similar flavor profile in recipes that call for tomatoes.

3. **Bananas:**
   - Swap bananas for lower-potassium fruits such as apples, berries, grapes, or peaches.
   - Opt for half a banana instead of a whole one to reduce potassium intake while still enjoying the flavor.

4. **Oranges and Orange Juice:**
   - Choose lower-potassium citrus fruits like clementines, tangerines, or mandarins as alternatives to oranges.
   - Replace orange juice with apple, cranberry, or grape juice, which have lower potassium content.

5. **Avocado:**
   - Substitute avocado with sliced cucumber, radishes, or lettuce in salads and sandwiches for a similar creamy texture.
   - Use hummus or low-fat cottage cheese as spreads or dips instead of avocado.

6. **Spinach:**
   - Replace spinach with lower-potassium leafy greens such as kale, Swiss chard, or romaine lettuce in salads, stir-fries, and soups.
   - Use cooked cabbage, bok choy, or green beans as alternatives to cooked spinach in recipes.

7. **Nuts and Seeds:**
    - Choose lower-potassium nuts and seeds such as almonds, pecans, pistachios, or sunflower seeds instead of high-potassium options like peanuts, cashews, or pumpkin seeds.
    - Limit portion sizes to small servings to manage potassium intake effectively.

8. **Beans and Legumes:**
    - Opt for lower-potassium beans such as green beans, wax beans, or black-eyed peas instead of high-potassium varieties like kidney beans, pinto beans, or black beans.
    - Rinse canned beans under cold water before use to reduce potassium content.

9. **Yogurt:**
    - Choose lower-potassium yogurt options such as Greek yogurt or strained yogurt with less potassium content compared to regular yogurt.
    - Opt for unsweetened almond milk or coconut milk yogurt as non-dairy alternatives with lower potassium levels.

10. **Tomato-Based Products:**
    - Replace tomato sauce, tomato paste, and tomato-based pasta sauces with alternatives made from vegetables like butternut squash, carrots, or beets for a similar texture and flavor profile.
    - Use herbs, spices, and garlic for added flavor in dishes traditionally made with tomato-based products.

Cooking Equipment and Tools for Kidney-Friendly Cooking

1. **Nonstick Cookware:** Nonstick pots and pans require less oil or fat for cooking, making them ideal for reducing added fats and oils in recipes. Choose high-quality nonstick cookware with durable coatings that are free of harmful chemicals like PFOA and PFAS.

2. **Stainless Steel Cookware:** Stainless steel pots and pans are durable, versatile, and easy to clean. They're suitable for cooking a variety of dishes, including soups, sauces, stir-fries, and pasta.

3. **Steamer Basket:** A steamer basket is an essential tool for steaming vegetables, fish, poultry, and grains. Steaming helps retain nutrients, texture, and flavor without the need for added fats or oils.

4. **Blender or Food Processor:** A blender or food processor is useful for pureeing soups, sauces, dips, and smoothies. Choose a high-powered blender or food processor with various speed settings and sharp blades for smooth and consistent results.

5. **Slow Cooker or Crockpot:** A slow cooker or crockpot is a convenient appliance for preparing kidney-friendly stews, soups, chili, and casseroles. Slow cooking allows flavors to develop over time while tenderizing tough cuts of meat and legumes.

6. **Grill or Grill Pan:** Grilling is a healthy cooking method that adds smoky flavor to meats, poultry, fish, and vegetables. Use an outdoor grill or stovetop grill pan to cook food without adding extra fats or oils.

7. **Vegetable Spiralizer:** A vegetable spiralizer is a handy tool for turning vegetables like zucchini, carrots, and cucumbers into noodles or "zoodles." Use spiralized vegetables as a low-carb, low-potassium alternative to pasta in kidney-friendly recipes.

8. **Digital Kitchen Scale:** A digital kitchen scale is essential for accurate portion control and measuring ingredients, especially for individuals with kidney disease who need to monitor nutrient intake closely.

9. **Citrus Juicer:** A citrus juicer or reamer is useful for extracting juice from lemons, limes, oranges, and grapefruits for use in marinades, dressings, sauces, and beverages.

10. **Herb Stripper:** An herb stripper is a handy tool for removing leaves from fresh herbs like thyme, rosemary, and parsley quickly and efficiently.

11. **Sharp Knives:** High-quality, sharp knives are essential for safe and efficient food preparation. Invest in a set of chef's knives, paring knives, and utility knives for slicing, dicing, and chopping ingredients with precision.

12. **Cutting Boards:** Choose cutting boards made from durable materials like wood, bamboo, or plastic for chopping fruits, vegetables, meats, and poultry. Use separate cutting boards for raw and cooked foods to prevent cross-contamination.

Chapter 5: Breakfast Recipes

Low-Sodium and Low-Phosphorus Breakfast Options

Spinach and Mushroom Breakfast Wrap:

Prep Time: 10 minutes **Cook Time:** 5 minutes **Servings:** 1

Ingredients:

- 1 whole wheat tortilla
- 2 eggs, scrambled
- 1/4 cup sliced mushrooms
- 1/4 cup chopped spinach
- 2 tablespoons shredded low-fat cheese
- Salt and pepper to taste

Instructions:

1. Heat a nonstick skillet over medium heat. Add sliced mushrooms and cook until softened.
2. Add chopped spinach to the skillet and cook until wilted. Season with salt and pepper.
3. Remove the vegetables from the skillet and set aside.
4. In the same skillet, scramble the eggs until cooked through.
5. Warm the whole wheat tortilla in the skillet or microwave for a few seconds.
6. Place the scrambled eggs, cooked vegetables, and shredded cheese in the center of the tortilla.
7. Fold the sides of the tortilla over the filling to form a wrap.
8. Serve hot with a side of fresh fruit or a small salad.

Nutritional Values (Approximate):

Calories: 300-350 kcal | Protein: 20-25 grams | Fat: 15-18 grams | Carbohydrates: 20-25 grams | Fiber: 3-5 grams | Sugars: 2-3 grams

Egg White Scramble with Vegetables:

Prep Time: 10 minutes   **Cook Time:** 5 minutes

Servings: 1

Ingredients:

- 3 egg whites
- 1/4 cup diced bell peppers
- 1/4 cup diced onions
- 1/4 cup diced tomatoes
- 1/4 cup chopped spinach
- 1 teaspoon olive oil
- Salt-free seasoning blend to taste

Instructions:

1. Heat olive oil in a nonstick skillet over medium heat.
2. Add diced bell peppers, onions, and tomatoes to the skillet and sauté until softened.
3. Add chopped spinach and cook until wilted.
4. Whisk the egg whites in a bowl and pour them over the cooked vegetables in the skillet.
5. Scramble the eggs until cooked through.
6. Season with salt-free seasoning blend to taste.
7. Serve hot with a side of whole grain toast or a small fruit salad.

Nutritional Values (Approximate, per serving): Calories: 150-200 kcal | Protein: 20-25 grams | Fat: 5-7 grams | Carbohydrates: 10-12 grams | Fiber: 2-3 grams | Sugars: 5-6 grams

Low-Sodium Cottage Cheese with Fresh Fruit:

Prep Time: 5 minutes   **Servings:** 1

Ingredients:

- 1/2 cup low-sodium cottage cheese
- 1/2 cup fresh fruit (such as sliced strawberries, blueberries, or peaches)
- 1 tablespoon chopped nuts (such as almonds or walnuts) (optional)

Instructions:

1. Place low-sodium cottage cheese in a serving bowl or dish.
2. Top with fresh fruit of your choice.
3. Sprinkle chopped nuts on top if desired.
4. Serve chilled or at room temperature.

Nutritional Values (Approximate):

Calories: 150-200 kcal | Protein: 15-20 grams | Fat: 5-7 grams | Carbohydrates: 15-20 grams | Fiber: 2-4 grams | Sugars: 10-15 grams

Oatmeal with Berries and Almond Milk:

- **Prep Time:** 5 minutes
- **Cook Time:** 5 minutes
- **Servings:** 1

Ingredients:

- 1/2 cup rolled oats (low-sodium)
- 1 cup unsweetened almond milk (low-sodium)
- 1/4 cup mixed berries (such as strawberries, blueberries, raspberries)
- 1 tablespoon chopped almonds (optional)
- Cinnamon to taste (optional)

Instructions:

1. In a small saucepan, bring almond milk to a boil over medium heat.
2. Stir in rolled oats and reduce heat to low. Cook for 3-5 minutes, stirring occasionally, until oats are cooked and the mixture thickens.

3. Remove from heat and let it sit for a minute to cool slightly.
4. Transfer oatmeal to a serving bowl and top with mixed berries and chopped almonds.
5. Sprinkle with cinnamon if desired.
6. Serve hot and enjoy.

Nutritional Values (Approximate):

Calories: 250-300 kcal | Protein: 8-10 grams | Fat: 8-10 grams | Carbohydrates: 35-40 grams | Fiber: 6-8 grams | Sugars: 5-8 grams

Protein-Rich Breakfast Ideas

Greek Yogurt Parfait:

Prep Time: 5 minutes   **Servings:** 1

Ingredients:

- 1/2 cup low-fat Greek yogurt
- 1/4 cup granola (low-sodium)
- 1/4 cup mixed berries (such as strawberries, blueberries, raspberries)
- 1 tablespoon honey or maple syrup (optional)

Instructions:

1. In a serving glass or bowl, layer Greek yogurt, granola, and mixed berries.
2. Drizzle honey or maple syrup on top for added sweetness if desired.
3. Repeat layers if making multiple servings.
4. Serve immediately as a nutritious and satisfying breakfast option.

Nutritional Values (Approximate):

Calories: 250-300 kcal | Protein: 15-18 grams | Fat: 5-7 grams | Carbohydrates: 35-40 grams | Fiber: 5-7 grams | Sugars: 15-20 grams

Egg and Veggie Breakfast Burrito:

Prep Time: 10 minutes **Cook Time:** 10 minutes **Servings:** 1

Ingredients:

- 2 eggs, scrambled
- 1 whole wheat tortilla
- 1/4 cup diced bell peppers
- 1/4 cup diced onions
- 1/4 cup chopped spinach
- 1/4 cup black beans, rinsed and drained
- 2 tablespoons shredded cheese
- Salsa or avocado for topping (optional)

Instructions:

1. In a nonstick skillet, heat olive oil over medium heat. Add diced bell peppers and onions, sauté until softened, about 3-4 minutes.
2. Add chopped spinach and black beans to the skillet, cook until spinach is wilted and beans are heated through, about 2 minutes.
3. Remove vegetables from the skillet and set aside.
4. In the same skillet, add a little more olive oil if needed, then pour in the scrambled eggs.
5. Cook eggs, stirring occasionally, until they are scrambled and cooked through, about 3-4 minutes.
6. Warm the whole wheat tortilla in the skillet or microwave.
7. Spoon the scrambled eggs and vegetable mixture onto the tortilla.
8. Sprinkle shredded cheese on top.
9. Roll up the tortilla to form a burrito.
10. Serve warm with salsa or sliced avocado if desired.

Nutritional Values (Approximate):

Calories: 350-400 kcal | Protein: 20-25 grams | Fat: 15-18 grams | Carbohydrates: 30-35 grams | Fiber: 5-7 grams | Sugars: 2-3 grams

Protein Smoothie:

Prep Time: 5 minutes **Servings:** 1

Ingredients:

- 1 scoop protein powder (whey, soy, or pea protein)
- 1 cup unsweetened almond milk or low-fat milk
- 1/2 banana
- 1/2 cup frozen berries (such as strawberries, blueberries, raspberries)
- 1 tablespoon nut butter (such as almond butter or peanut butter)
- Handful of spinach (optional)
- Ice cubes (optional)

Instructions:

1. In a blender, combine protein powder, almond milk, banana, frozen berries, nut butter, and spinach.
2. Blend until smooth and creamy.
3. Add ice cubes if desired for a colder texture.
4. Pour into a glass and enjoy immediately.

Nutritional Values (Approximate):

Calories: 300-350 kcal | Protein: 20-25 grams | Fat: 10-15 grams | Carbohydrates: 25-30 grams | Fiber: 5-7 grams | Sugars: 10-15 grams

Protein Pancakes

Prep Time: 10 minutes **Cook Time:** 10 minutes **Servings:** 2-3 pancakes

Ingredients:

- 1/2 cup oats
- 1/2 cup low-fat cottage cheese
- 2 eggs
- 1/2 teaspoon vanilla extract
- 1/2 teaspoon cinnamon
- Cooking spray or butter for greasing the pan

Instructions:

1. In a blender, combine oats, cottage cheese, eggs, vanilla extract, and cinnamon. Blend until smooth.
2. Heat a nonstick skillet or griddle over medium heat and lightly grease with cooking spray or butter.
3. Pour batter onto the skillet to form pancakes of desired size.
4. Cook until bubbles form on the surface, then flip and cook until golden brown on the other side.
5. Repeat with the remaining batter.
6. Serve hot with your favorite toppings such as Greek yogurt, berries, or nut butter.

Nutritional Values (Approximate, per serving - 2 pancakes): Calories: 250-300 kcal | Protein: 20-25 grams | Fat: 10-12 grams | Carbohydrates: 20-25 grams | Fiber: 3-5 grams | Sugars: 2-3 grams

Creative and Nutritious Smoothie Recipes

Green Power Smoothie:

Prep Time: 5 minutes **Servings:** 1

Ingredients:

- 1 cup spinach
- 1/2 ripe avocado
- 1/2 banana
- 1 scoop vanilla protein powder
- 1 tablespoon chia seeds
- 1 cup unsweetened almond milk
- Ice cubes (optional)

Instructions:

1. In a blender, combine spinach, avocado, banana, protein powder, chia seeds, and almond milk.
2. Blend until smooth and creamy.
3. Add ice cubes if desired for a colder texture.
4. Pour into a glass and enjoy this nutrient-packed smoothie.

Nutritional Values (Approximate):

Calories: 300-350 kcal | Protein: 25-30 grams | Fat: 15-18 grams | Carbohydrates: 20-25 grams | Fiber: 10-12 grams | Sugars: 5-7 grams

Berry Blast Smoothie:

Prep Time: 5 minutes **Servings:** 1

Ingredients:

- 1/2 cup mixed berries (such as strawberries, blueberries, raspberries)
- 1/2 cup plain Greek yogurt
- 1 scoop vanilla protein powder
- 1 tablespoon almond butter
- 1 teaspoon honey or maple syrup (optional)
- 1 cup unsweetened almond milk
- Ice cubes (optional)

Instructions:

1. In a blender, combine mixed berries, Greek yogurt, protein powder, almond butter, honey or maple syrup, and almond milk.
2. Blend until smooth and well combined.
3. Add ice cubes if desired for a colder texture.
4. Pour into a glass and enjoy this delicious and nutritious berry smoothie.

Nutritional Values (Approximate):

Calories: 300-350 kcal | Protein: 25-30 grams | Fat: 10-12 grams | Carbohydrates: 20-25 grams | Fiber: 5-7 grams | Sugars: 10-12 grams

Tropical Paradise Smoothie:

Prep Time: 5 minutes **Servings:** 1

Ingredients:

- 1/2 cup frozen pineapple chunks
- 1/2 cup frozen mango chunks
- 1/2 ripe banana
- 1 scoop coconut-flavored protein powder
- 1 tablespoon shredded coconut
- 1 cup coconut water or unsweetened almond milk
- Ice cubes (optional)

Instructions:

1. In a blender, combine frozen pineapple chunks, frozen mango chunks, banana, protein powder, shredded coconut, and coconut water or almond milk.
2. Blend until smooth and creamy.
3. Add ice cubes if desired for a colder texture.
4. Pour into a glass and enjoy this tropical-inspired smoothie bursting with flavor.

Nutritional Values (Approximate):

Calories: 250-300 kcal | Protein: 20-25 grams | Fat: 5-7 grams | Carbohydrates: 30-35 grams | Fiber: 5-7 grams | Sugars: 20-25 grams

Chapter 6

Lunch and Dinner Recipes

Kidney-Friendly Main Dishes with Lean Protein Sources

Baked Lemon Herb Salmon:

Prep Time: 10 minutes **Cook Time:** 15 minutes **Servings:** 4

Ingredients:

- 4 salmon fillets (about 6 ounces each)
- 2 tablespoons olive oil
- 2 cloves garlic, minced
- 1 tablespoon fresh lemon juice
- 1 teaspoon lemon zest
- 1 teaspoon dried oregano
- 1 teaspoon dried thyme
- Salt and pepper to taste
- Lemon slices for garnish
- Fresh parsley for garnish

Instructions:

1. Preheat oven to 400°F (200°C). Line a baking sheet with parchment paper.
2. In a small bowl, whisk together olive oil, minced garlic, lemon juice, lemon zest, oregano, thyme, salt, and pepper.
3. Place salmon fillets on the prepared baking sheet. Brush each fillet with the lemon herb mixture, coating evenly.
4. Bake in the preheated oven for 12-15 minutes, or until salmon flakes easily with a fork.
5. Remove from the oven and garnish with lemon slices and fresh parsley before serving.

Nutritional Values (Approximate):

Calories: 300-350 kcal | Protein: 30-35 grams | Fat: 15-18 grams | Carbohydrates: 1-2 grams | Fiber: 0 grams | Sugars: 0 grams

Grilled Chicken Salad:

Prep Time: 15 minutes **Cook Time:** 10 minutes **Servings:** 2

Ingredients:

- 2 boneless, skinless chicken breasts
- 4 cups mixed greens (such as lettuce, spinach, arugula)
- 1 cup cherry tomatoes, halved
- 1/2 cucumber, sliced
- 1/4 red onion, thinly sliced
- 1/4 cup crumbled feta cheese
- 2 tablespoons olive oil
- 1 tablespoon balsamic vinegar
- Salt and pepper to taste

Instructions:

1. Preheat grill to medium-high heat.
2. Season chicken breasts with salt and pepper.
3. Grill chicken for 4-5 minutes per side, or until cooked through and no longer pink in the center.
4. In a large bowl, combine mixed greens, cherry tomatoes, cucumber, red onion, and feta cheese.
5. In a small bowl, whisk together olive oil and balsamic vinegar to make the dressing.
6. Slice grilled chicken and add to the salad.
7. Drizzle dressing over the salad and toss to combine.
8. Divide salad between plates and serve.

Nutritional Values (Approximate):

Calories: 300-350 kcal | Protein: 30-35 grams | Fat: 15-18 grams | Carbohydrates: 10-12 grams | Fiber: 3-5 grams | Sugars: 5-7 grams

Quinoa Stuffed Bell Peppers:

Prep Time: 20 minutes **Cook Time:** 30 minutes **Servings:** 4

Ingredients:

- 4 bell peppers, any color
- 1 cup quinoa, rinsed
- 2 cups vegetable broth or water
- 1 can (15 oz) black beans, rinsed and drained
- 1 cup corn kernels
- 1 cup diced tomatoes
- 1/2 cup diced red onion
- 1/4 cup chopped fresh cilantro
- 1 teaspoon ground cumin
- 1/2 teaspoon chili powder
- Salt and pepper to taste
- 1/2 cup shredded cheese (optional)

Instructions:

1. Preheat oven to 375°F (190°C).
2. Cut the tops off the bell peppers and remove the seeds and membranes.
3. In a medium saucepan, combine quinoa and vegetable broth. Bring to a boil, then reduce heat to low, cover, and simmer for 15 minutes, or until quinoa is cooked and liquid is absorbed.
4. In a large bowl, combine cooked quinoa, black beans, corn, diced tomatoes, red onion, cilantro, cumin, chili powder, salt, and pepper. Mix well.
5. Stuff each bell pepper with the quinoa mixture.
6. Place stuffed peppers in a baking dish. If using cheese, sprinkle it over the tops of the peppers.
7. Cover the baking dish with foil and bake for 25-30 minutes, or until peppers are tender.
8. Remove foil and bake for an additional 5 minutes, or until cheese is melted and bubbly (if using).
9. Serve hot.

Nutritional Values (Approximate):

Calories: 300-350 kcal | Protein: 10-12 grams | Fat: 5-7 grams | Carbohydrates: 55-60 grams | Fiber: 10-12 grams | Sugars: 5-7 grams

Delicious Side Dishes with Controlled Sodium and Potassium

Roasted Garlic Mashed Cauliflower:

Prep Time: 10 minutes **Cook Time:** 25 minutes **Servings:** 4

Ingredients:

- 1 head cauliflower, cut into florets
- 2 cloves garlic, minced
- 1 tablespoon olive oil
- Salt and pepper to taste
- Chopped fresh chives for garnish (optional)

Instructions:

1. Preheat oven to 400°F (200°C). Line a baking sheet with parchment paper.
2. In a large bowl, toss cauliflower florets with minced garlic, olive oil, salt, and pepper until evenly coated.
3. Spread cauliflower in a single layer on the prepared baking sheet.
4. Roast in the preheated oven for 20-25 minutes, or until cauliflower is tender and lightly golden brown, stirring halfway through.
5. Remove from the oven and transfer roasted cauliflower to a food processor.
6. Pulse until cauliflower is mashed to desired consistency.
7. Season with additional salt and pepper if needed.
8. Garnish with chopped fresh chives before serving.

Nutritional Values (Approximate):

Calories: 50-60 kcal | Protein: 2-3 grams | Fat: 2-3 grams | Carbohydrates: 5-7 grams | Fiber: 2-3 grams | Sugars: 2-3 grams

Lemon Herb Quinoa Salad:

Prep Time: 10 minutes **Cook Time:** 15 minutes **Servings:** 4

Ingredients:

- 1 cup quinoa, rinsed
- 2 cups low-sodium vegetable broth or water
- 1/4 cup chopped fresh parsley
- 1/4 cup chopped fresh cilantro
- 2 tablespoons chopped fresh dill
- 2 tablespoons olive oil
- 2 tablespoons fresh lemon juice
- 1 teaspoon lemon zest
- Salt and pepper to taste

Instructions:

1. In a medium saucepan, bring vegetable broth or water to a boil.
2. Stir in quinoa, reduce heat to low, cover, and simmer for 15 minutes, or until quinoa is cooked and liquid is absorbed.
3. Fluff quinoa with a fork and transfer to a large bowl.
4. Add chopped parsley, cilantro, and dill to the quinoa.
5. In a small bowl, whisk together olive oil, lemon juice, lemon zest, salt, and pepper to make the dressing.
6. Pour dressing over the quinoa and herbs, and toss to combine.
7. Serve the lemon herb quinoa salad warm or chilled.

Nutritional Values (Approximate):

Calories: 150-200 kcal | Protein: 4-5 grams | Fat: 7-9 grams | Carbohydrates: 20-25 grams | Fiber: 3-4 grams | Sugars: 1-2 grams

Vegetarian and Vegan Options for Balanced Nutrition

Lentil and Vegetable Stir-Fry:

Prep Time: 15 minutes **Cook Time:** 20 minutes **Servings:** 4

Ingredients:

- 1 cup dry lentils, rinsed and drained
- 2 cups vegetable broth or water
- 2 tablespoons olive oil
- 2 cloves garlic, minced
- 1 onion, diced
- 2 carrots, sliced
- 1 bell pepper, sliced
- 1 cup broccoli florets
- 1 cup snap peas
- 1/4 cup soy sauce (or tamari for gluten-free option)
- 1 tablespoon rice vinegar
- 1 tablespoon maple syrup
- 1 teaspoon sesame oil (optional)
- Cooked brown rice or quinoa for serving

Instructions:

1. In a medium saucepan, combine lentils and vegetable broth or water. Bring to a boil, then reduce heat to low, cover, and simmer for 15-20 minutes, or until lentils are tender.
2. In a large skillet or wok, heat olive oil over medium heat. Add minced garlic and diced onion, and cook until softened, about 3-4 minutes.
3. Add sliced carrots, bell pepper, broccoli florets, and snap peas to the skillet. Stir-fry for 5-6 minutes, or until vegetables are tender-crisp.
4. In a small bowl, whisk together soy sauce, rice vinegar, maple syrup, and sesame oil (if using).
5. Add cooked lentils and the soy sauce mixture to the skillet with the vegetables. Stir well to combine and heat through.
6. Serve the lentil and vegetable stir-fry over cooked brown rice or quinoa.

Nutritional Values (Approximate):

Calories: 250-300 kcal | Protein: 12-15 grams | Fat: 7-9 grams | Carbohydrates: 35-40 grams | Fiber: 10-12 grams | Sugars: 8-10 grams

Chickpea and Spinach Curry:

Prep Time: 10 minutes **Cook Time:** 20 minutes **Servings:** 4

Ingredients:

- 2 tablespoons olive oil
- 1 onion, diced
- 2 cloves garlic, minced
- 1 tablespoon fresh ginger, grated
- 1 tablespoon curry powder
- 1 teaspoon ground cumin
- 1 teaspoon ground coriander
- 1/2 teaspoon turmeric powder
- 1/4 teaspoon cayenne pepper (optional)
- 1 can (15 oz) chickpeas, rinsed and drained
- 1 can (14 oz) diced tomatoes
- 2 cups fresh spinach leaves
- Salt and pepper to taste
- Cooked brown rice or quinoa for serving

Instructions:

1. In a large skillet or pot, heat olive oil over medium heat. Add diced onion and cook until translucent, about 3-4 minutes.
2. Add minced garlic and grated ginger to the skillet, and cook for an additional 1-2 minutes, until fragrant.
3. Stir in curry powder, cumin, coriander, turmeric, and cayenne pepper (if using), and cook for another minute.
4. Add chickpeas and diced tomatoes to the skillet, and bring to a simmer. Cook for 10-15 minutes, stirring occasionally, until the sauce thickens slightly.
5. Add fresh spinach leaves to the skillet and cook until wilted, about 2-3 minutes.
6. Season with salt and pepper to taste.
7. Serve the chickpea and spinach curry over cooked brown rice or quinoa.

Nutritional Values (Approximate): Calories: 200-250 kcal | Protein: 8-10 grams | Fat: 7-9 grams | Carbohydrates: 25-30 grams | Fiber: 8-10 grams | Sugars: 5-7 grams

One-Pot Meals for Easy Preparation and Cleanup

One-Pot Chicken and Rice:

Prep Time: 10 minutes
Cook Time: 30 minutes
Servings: 4

Ingredients:

- 4 boneless, skinless chicken thighs
- 1 cup long-grain white rice
- 2 cups low-sodium chicken broth
- 1 onion, chopped
- 2 cloves garlic, minced
- 1 bell pepper, diced
- 1 cup diced tomatoes
- 1 teaspoon dried thyme
- 1 teaspoon paprika
- Salt and pepper to taste
- Fresh parsley for garnish

Instructions:

1. Season the chicken thighs with salt, pepper, and paprika.
2. In a large skillet or pot, heat some olive oil over medium-high heat. Add the chicken thighs and cook until browned on both sides, about 5 minutes per side. Remove the chicken and set it aside.
3. In the same skillet, add the chopped onion, minced garlic, and diced bell pepper. Cook until softened, about 3-4 minutes.
4. Stir in the rice, diced tomatoes, dried thyme, and chicken broth. Bring the mixture to a boil.
5. Reduce the heat to low, return the chicken thighs to the skillet, cover, and simmer for 20 minutes, or until the rice is cooked and the chicken is cooked through.
6. Garnish with fresh parsley before serving.

Nutritional Values (Approximate):

Calories: 250-300 kcal | Protein: 20-25 grams | Fat: 8-10 grams | Carbohydrates: 20-25 grams | Fiber: 2-3 grams | Sugars: 3-4 grams

One-Pot Vegetable Pasta Primavera:

Prep Time: 10 minutes
Cook Time: 20 minutes
Servings: 4

Ingredients:

- 8 oz penne pasta
- 2 cups chopped mixed vegetables (such as bell peppers, zucchini, cherry tomatoes, broccoli)
- 2 cloves garlic, minced
- 4 cups low-sodium vegetable broth
- 1/2 cup grated Parmesan cheese (optional)
- 2 tablespoons olive oil
- Salt and pepper to taste
- Fresh basil for garnish

Instructions:

1. In a large pot, heat olive oil over medium heat. Add minced garlic and cook until fragrant, about 1 minute.
2. Add chopped mixed vegetables to the pot and cook for 3-4 minutes, stirring occasionally.
3. Stir in penne pasta and vegetable broth. Bring to a boil.
4. Reduce heat to low, cover, and simmer for 12-15 minutes, or until pasta is cooked and most of the liquid is absorbed.
5. If using, stir in grated Parmesan cheese until melted and well combined.
6. Season with salt and pepper to taste.
7. Garnish with fresh basil before serving.

Nutritional Values (Approximate):

Calories: 300-350 kcal | Protein: 8-10 grams | Fat: 6-8 grams | Carbohydrates: 50-60 grams | Fiber: 5-7 grams | Sugars: 5-7 grams

Chapter 7: Snacks and Appetizers

Nutrient-Dense Snack Ideas for Kidney Health

Greek Yogurt with Berries and Almonds:

Prep Time: 5 minutes
Servings: 1

Ingredients:

- 1/2 cup Greek yogurt
- 1/4 cup mixed berries (such as strawberries, blueberries, raspberries)
- 1 tablespoon sliced almonds

Instructions:

1. In a serving bowl, place Greek yogurt.
2. Top with mixed berries and sliced almonds.
3. Serve immediately.

Nutritional Values (Approximate):

Calories: 150-200 kcal | Protein: 12-15 grams | Fat: 5-7 grams | Carbohydrates: 15-20 grams | Fiber: 3-5 grams | Sugars: 8-10 grams

Hummus and Veggie Sticks:

Prep Time: 10 minutes
Servings: 2

Ingredients:

- 1/2 cup hummus
- 2 carrots, sliced into sticks
- 2 celery stalks, sliced into sticks
- 1 cucumber, sliced into sticks

Instructions:

1. Place hummus in a serving bowl.
2. Arrange carrot, celery, and cucumber sticks around the hummus.
3. Serve immediately.

Nutritional Values (Approximate):

Calories: 200-250 kcal | Protein: 8-10 grams | Fat: 10-12 grams | Carbohydrates: 20-25 grams | Fiber: 8-10 grams | Sugars: 5-7 grams

Hard-Boiled Eggs with Whole Grain Crackers:

Prep Time: 10 minutes (for boiling eggs)
Servings: 2

Ingredients:

- 4 hard-boiled eggs
- 8 whole grain crackers

Instructions:

1. Peel the hard-boiled eggs and slice them in half.
2. Place the hard-boiled eggs and whole grain crackers on a serving plate.
3. Serve immediately.

Nutritional Values (Approximate):

Calories: 250-300 kcal | Protein: 16-20 grams | Fat: 12-15 grams | Carbohydrates: 16-20 grams | Fiber: 3-5 grams | Sugars: 1-2 grams

Cottage Cheese with Pineapple:

Prep Time: 5 minutes
Servings: 1

Ingredients:

- 1/2 cup cottage cheese
- 1/2 cup pineapple chunks (fresh or canned, drained)

Instructions:

1. Place cottage cheese in a serving bowl.
2. Top with pineapple chunks.
3. Serve immediately.

Nutritional Values (Approximate):

Calories: 150-200 kcal | Protein: 15-20 grams | Fat: 2-4 grams | Carbohydrates: 20-25 grams | Fiber: 1-2 grams | Sugars: 15-20 grams

Trail Mix with Nuts and Dried Fruit:

Prep Time: 5 minutes
Servings: 2

Ingredients:

- 1/2 cup mixed nuts (such as almonds, cashews, walnuts)
- 1/4 cup dried fruit (such as raisins, cranberries, apricots)

Instructions:

1. Mix together mixed nuts and dried fruit in a bowl.
2. Serve immediately or store in an airtight container for later use.

Nutritional Values (Approximate):

Calories: 250-300 kcal | Protein: 6-8 grams | Fat: 15-20 grams | Carbohydrates: 20-25 grams | Fiber: 3-5 grams | Sugars: 10-15 grams

Avocado Toast with Tomato Slices:

Prep Time: 5 minutes
Servings: 1

Ingredients:

- 1 ripe avocado
- 2 slices whole grain bread, toasted
- 1 medium tomato, sliced
- Salt and pepper to taste
- Optional toppings: red pepper flakes, sesame seeds, fresh herbs

Instructions:

1. Cut the ripe avocado in half, remove the pit, and scoop out the flesh into a bowl.
2. Mash the avocado with a fork until smooth or chunky, according to preference.
3. Spread the mashed avocado evenly onto the toasted whole grain bread slices.
4. Top the avocado toast with tomato slices.
5. Season with salt, pepper, and any optional toppings.
6. Serve immediately.

Nutritional Values (Approximate):

Calories: 250-300 kcal | Protein: 7-9 grams | Fat: 15-18 grams | Carbohydrates: 25-30 grams | Fiber: 8-10 grams | Sugars: 2-3 grams

Yogurt and Fruit Parfait:

Prep Time: 5 minutes
Servings: 1

Ingredients:

- 1/2 cup Greek yogurt
- 1/2 cup mixed fresh fruits (such as berries, sliced banana, diced mango)
- 1/4 cup granola
- Optional toppings: honey, nuts, seeds

Instructions:

1. In a serving glass or bowl, layer Greek yogurt, mixed fresh fruits, and granola.
2. Repeat the layers if desired.
3. Drizzle with honey and sprinkle with nuts or seeds if using.
4. Serve immediately.

Nutritional Values (Approximate):

Calories: 250-300 kcal | Protein: 15-18 grams | Fat: 6-8 grams | Carbohydrates: 35-40 grams | Fiber: 5-7 grams | Sugars: 15-20 grams

Mini Vegetable Frittatas:

Prep Time: 15 minutes **Cook Time:** 20 minutes
Servings: 12 mini frittatas

Ingredients:

- 6 large eggs
- 1/4 cup milk or unsweetened almond milk
- 1/2 cup chopped mixed vegetables (such as bell peppers, spinach, onions)
- 1/4 cup shredded low-fat cheese
- Salt and pepper to taste
- Cooking spray

Instructions:

1. Preheat the oven to 350°F (175°C). Grease a muffin tin with cooking spray.
2. In a mixing bowl, whisk together eggs and milk. Season with salt and pepper.
3. Divide the chopped mixed vegetables evenly among the muffin cups.
4. Pour the egg mixture over the vegetables, filling each muffin cup about 3/4 full.
5. Sprinkle shredded cheese on top of each frittata.
6. Bake in the preheated oven for 18-20 minutes, or until the frittatas are set and lightly golden on top.
7. Allow the frittatas to cool for a few minutes before removing them from the muffin tin.
8. Serve warm or at room temperature.

Nutritional Values (Approximate):

Calories: 50-60 kcal | Protein: 4-5 grams | Fat: 3-4 grams | Carbohydrates: 1-2 grams | Fiber: 0-1 grams | Sugars: 0 grams

Stuffed Mushrooms with Quinoa and Spinach:

Prep Time: 20 minutes **Cook Time:** 25 minutes
Servings: 12 stuffed mushrooms

Ingredients:

- 12 large mushrooms, stems removed and finely chopped
- 1/2 cup cooked quinoa
- 1/2 cup chopped spinach
- 1/4 cup diced onion
- 2 cloves garlic, minced
- 1/4 cup shredded low-fat cheese
- Salt and pepper to taste
- Cooking spray

Instructions:

1. Preheat the oven to 375°F (190°C). Line a baking sheet with parchment paper and lightly grease with cooking spray.
2. In a skillet, heat some cooking spray over medium heat. Add chopped mushroom stems, diced onion, and minced garlic. Cook until softened, about 3-4 minutes.
3. Stir in cooked quinoa and chopped spinach. Cook for another 2-3 minutes, until the spinach wilts.
4. Season the quinoa mixture with salt and pepper to taste.
5. Spoon the quinoa mixture into the mushroom caps, filling each one generously.
6. Place the stuffed mushrooms on the prepared baking sheet.
7. Sprinkle shredded cheese over the top of each stuffed mushroom.
8. Bake in the preheated oven for 20-25 minutes, or until the mushrooms are tender and the cheese is melted and golden.
9. Allow the stuffed mushrooms to cool for a few minutes before serving.

Nutritional Values (Approximate):

Calories: 40-50 kcal | Protein: 2-3 grams | Fat: 1-2 grams | Carbohydrates: 5-6 grams | Fiber: 1-2 grams | Sugars: 1-2 grams

Portable Snacks for On-the-Go Convenience

Homemade Trail Mix:

Prep Time: 5 minutes
Servings: 4

Ingredients:

- 1/2 cup mixed nuts (such as almonds, cashews, walnuts)
- 1/4 cup dried fruit (such as raisins, cranberries, apricots)
- 1/4 cup whole grain cereal or pretzel pieces
- 2 tablespoons dark chocolate chips or chunks (optional)

Instructions:

1. Mix together mixed nuts, dried fruit, whole grain cereal or pretzel pieces, and dark chocolate chips or chunks in a bowl.
2. Divide the trail mix into individual portion-sized containers or resealable bags.
3. Store in a cool, dry place or take it with you for on-the-go snacking.

Nutritional Values (Approximate):

Calories: 150-200 kcal | Protein: 4-6 grams | Fat: 8-10 grams | Carbohydrates: 15-20 grams | Fiber: 2-4 grams | Sugars: 8-10 grams

Greek Yogurt Cups with Berries:

Prep Time: 5 minutes
Servings: 1

Ingredients:

- 1/2 cup Greek yogurt
- 1/4 cup mixed berries (such as strawberries, blueberries, raspberries)
- 1 tablespoon honey or maple syrup (optional)
- Optional toppings: granola, nuts, seeds

Instructions:

1. Place Greek yogurt in a portable container with a lid.
2. Top the Greek yogurt with mixed berries.
3. Drizzle with honey or maple syrup if using.
4. Optionally, sprinkle with granola, nuts, or seeds for added crunch and flavor.
5. Seal the container and keep it refrigerated until ready to eat.

Nutritional Values (Approximate):

Calories: 150-200 kcal | Protein: 10-12 grams | Fat: 3-5 grams | Carbohydrates: 20-25 grams | Fiber: 2-4 grams | Sugars: 15-20 grams

Hummus and Veggie Sticks

Prep Time: 10 minutes
Servings: 2

Ingredients:

- 1/2 cup hummus
- 2 medium carrots, cut into sticks
- 2 celery stalks, cut into sticks
- 1/2 bell pepper, sliced
- 1/2 cucumber, sliced
- Optional: cherry tomatoes, snap peas, radishes

Instructions:

1. Place hummus in a portable container with a lid.
2. Arrange the veggie sticks and slices in another container or compartmentalized snack box.
3. Keep refrigerated until ready to eat.
4. Dip the veggie sticks into the hummus for a nutritious and satisfying snack.

Nutritional Values (Approximate):

Calories: 150-200 kcal | Protein: 5-7 grams | Fat: 8-10 grams | Carbohydrates: 15-20 grams | Fiber: 5-7 grams | Sugars: 3-5 grams

Chapter 8: Desserts and Sweet Treats

Banana Oatmeal Cookies:

Prep Time: 10 minutes
Cook Time: 15 minutes
Servings: 12 cookies

Ingredients:

- 2 ripe bananas, mashed
- 1 cup rolled oats
- 1/4 cup raisins or dried cranberries
- 1/4 cup chopped nuts (such as walnuts or almonds)
- 1/4 teaspoon cinnamon
- Optional: 1 tablespoon honey or maple syrup for added sweetness

Instructions:

1. Preheat the oven to 350°F (175°C). Line a baking sheet with parchment paper.
2. In a mixing bowl, combine mashed bananas, rolled oats, raisins or dried cranberries, chopped nuts, cinnamon, and optional honey or maple syrup. Mix until well combined.
3. Scoop spoonfuls of the cookie dough onto the prepared baking sheet, spacing them apart.
4. Flatten each cookie slightly with the back of a spoon or fork.
5. Bake in the preheated oven for 15 minutes, or until the cookies are golden brown and firm to the touch.
6. Allow the cookies to cool on the baking sheet for a few minutes before transferring them to a wire rack to cool completely.

Nutritional Values (Approximate):

Calories: 70-80 kcal | Protein: 2-3 grams | Fat: 2-3 grams | Carbohydrates: 12-15 grams | Fiber: 2-3 grams | Sugars: 5-7 grams

Frozen Yogurt Bark with Fruit:

Prep Time: 10 minutes
Freeze Time: 2 hours
Servings: 6 servings

Ingredients:

- 2 cups Greek yogurt (plain or flavored)
- 1 cup mixed fresh fruit (such as berries, sliced kiwi, diced mango)
- 2 tablespoons honey or maple syrup
- 1/4 cup granola or chopped nuts (optional)

Instructions:

1. Line a baking sheet with parchment paper.
2. In a mixing bowl, combine Greek yogurt and honey or maple syrup. Stir until smooth.
3. Spread the Greek yogurt mixture evenly onto the prepared baking sheet, about 1/4 inch thick.
4. Sprinkle mixed fresh fruit and granola or chopped nuts evenly over the yogurt layer.
5. Place the baking sheet in the freezer and freeze for at least 2 hours, or until the yogurt bark is frozen solid.
6. Once frozen, break the yogurt bark into pieces.
7. Serve immediately as a refreshing frozen treat.

Nutritional Values (Approximate):

Calories: 100-120 kcal | Protein: 6-8 grams | Fat: 2-3 grams | Carbohydrates: 15-20 grams | Fiber: 1-2 grams | Sugars: 10-12 grams

Baked Apples with Cinnamon and Nuts:

Prep Time: 10 minutes
Cook Time: 30 minutes
Servings: 4 servings

Ingredients:

- 4 apples (such as Granny Smith or Honeycrisp)
- 1/4 cup chopped nuts (such as walnuts or pecans)
- 2 tablespoons honey or maple syrup
- 1 teaspoon ground cinnamon
- Optional toppings: Greek yogurt, whipped cream, or vanilla ice cream

Instructions:

1. Preheat the oven to 375°F (190°C). Grease a baking dish with cooking spray or butter.
2. Core the apples and remove the seeds, leaving the bottoms intact.
3. Place the cored apples in the prepared baking dish.
4. In a small bowl, mix together chopped nuts, honey or maple syrup, and ground cinnamon.
5. Stuff each apple with the nut mixture, filling the centers evenly.
6. Cover the baking dish with aluminum foil and bake in the preheated oven for 20 minutes.
7. Remove the foil and bake for an additional 10 minutes, or until the apples are tender and the tops are golden brown.
8. Serve the baked apples warm, optionally topped with Greek yogurt, whipped cream, or vanilla ice cream.

Nutritional Values (Approximate):

Calories: 150-200 kcal | Protein: 2-3 grams | Fat: 5-7 grams | Carbohydrates: 25-30 grams | Fiber: 4-5 grams | Sugars: 20-25 grams

Low-Phosphorus Dessert Recipes for Indulgence without Compromise

Low-Phosphorus Chocolate Chia Pudding:

Prep Time: 5 minutes
Chill Time: 2 hours
Servings: 4

Ingredients:

- 1/4 cup chia seeds
- 1 cup unsweetened almond milk or low-phosphorus milk alternative
- 2 tablespoons unsweetened cocoa powder
- 2 tablespoons honey or maple syrup (optional, adjust to taste)
- 1/2 teaspoon vanilla extract
- Fresh berries or sliced fruit for topping (optional)

Instructions:

1. In a mixing bowl, combine chia seeds, unsweetened almond milk, cocoa powder, honey or maple syrup (if using), and vanilla extract. Stir until well combined.
2. Let the mixture sit for 5 minutes, then stir again to prevent clumping.
3. Cover the bowl and refrigerate for at least 2 hours, or preferably overnight, to allow the chia seeds to thicken and absorb the liquid.
4. Once the pudding has thickened to your desired consistency, give it a final stir.
5. Serve the chocolate chia pudding chilled, topped with fresh berries or sliced fruit if desired.

Nutritional Values (Approximate):

Calories: 100-120 kcal | Protein: 3-4 grams | Fat: 5-6 grams | Carbohydrates: 10-12 grams | Fiber: 5-6 grams | Sugars: 4-5 grams

Low-Phosphorus Berry Sorbet:

Prep Time: 10 minutes
Chill Time: 4 hours
Servings: 4

Ingredients:

- 2 cups mixed berries (such as strawberries, blueberries, raspberries)
- 1/4 cup water
- 2 tablespoons honey or maple syrup (optional, adjust to taste)
- 1 tablespoon lemon juice

Instructions:

1. Place mixed berries, water, honey or maple syrup (if using), and lemon juice in a blender or food processor.
2. Blend until smooth and well combined.
3. Taste the mixture and adjust sweetness if needed by adding more honey or maple syrup.
4. Pour the berry mixture into a shallow dish or baking pan.
5. Cover the dish or pan with plastic wrap and place it in the freezer.
6. Freeze for about 2 hours, then remove from the freezer and use a fork to break up any ice crystals that have formed.
7. Return the sorbet to the freezer and continue to freeze for another 2 hours, or until firm.
8. Serve the low-phosphorus berry sorbet scooped into bowls or glasses.

Nutritional Values (Approximate):

Calories: 50-70 kcal | Protein: 1-2 grams | Fat: 0 grams | Carbohydrates: 12-15 grams | Fiber: 2-3 grams | Sugars: 8-10 grams

Low-Phosphorus Coconut Milk Rice Pudding:

Prep Time: 5 minutes
Cook Time: 30 minutes
Chill Time: 2 hours
Servings: 4

Ingredients:

- 1/2 cup Arborio rice or short-grain rice
- 1 can (13.5 oz) coconut milk
- 1/4 cup honey or maple syrup (adjust to taste)
- 1 teaspoon vanilla extract
- Ground cinnamon or nutmeg for garnish (optional)

Instructions:

1. In a medium saucepan, combine Arborio rice, coconut milk, honey or maple syrup, and vanilla extract.
2. Bring the mixture to a gentle boil over medium heat, then reduce the heat to low and simmer, stirring occasionally, for 25-30 minutes, or until the rice is cooked and the mixture has thickened.
3. Remove the rice pudding from the heat and let it cool slightly.
4. Transfer the rice pudding to a serving dish or individual bowls.
5. Cover the rice pudding with plastic wrap, ensuring the wrap touches the surface of the pudding to prevent a skin from forming.
6. Chill the rice pudding in the refrigerator for at least 2 hours, or until cold.
7. Before serving, sprinkle ground cinnamon or nutmeg on top for added flavor if desired.

Nutritional Values (Approximate):

Calories: 250-300 kcal | Protein: 3-4 grams | Fat: 10-12 grams | Carbohydrates: 35-40 grams | Fiber: 1-2 grams | Sugars: 12-15 grams

Fruit-Based Desserts with Controlled Potassium

Low-Potassium Mango Sorbet:

Prep Time: 10 minutes
Chill Time: 4 hours
Servings: 4

Ingredients:

- 2 ripe mangoes, peeled and diced
- 1 tablespoon lemon juice
- 2 tablespoons honey or maple syrup (optional)
- 1/4 cup water

Instructions:

1. Place diced mangoes, lemon juice, honey or maple syrup (if using), and water in a blender or food processor.
2. Blend until smooth and well combined.
3. Taste the mixture and adjust sweetness if needed by adding more honey or maple syrup.
4. Pour the mango mixture into a shallow dish or baking pan.
5. Cover the dish or pan with plastic wrap and place it in the freezer.
6. Freeze for about 2 hours, then remove from the freezer and use a fork to break up any ice crystals that have formed.
7. Return the sorbet to the freezer and continue to freeze for another 2 hours, or until firm.
8. Serve the low-potassium mango sorbet scooped into bowls or glasses.

Nutritional Values (Approximate):

Calories: 70-90 kcal | Protein: 1 gram | Fat: 0 grams | Carbohydrates: 18-20 grams | Fiber: 2-3 grams | Sugars: 15-18 grams

Low-Potassium Berry Compote:

Prep Time: 5 minutes
Cook Time: 10 minutes
Servings: 4

Ingredients:

- 2 cups mixed berries (such as strawberries, blueberries, raspberries)
- 2 tablespoons honey or maple syrup
- 1 tablespoon lemon juice
- 1/2 teaspoon vanilla extract
- 1/4 cup water

Instructions:

1. In a saucepan, combine mixed berries, honey or maple syrup, lemon juice, vanilla extract, and water.
2. Bring the mixture to a simmer over medium heat, stirring occasionally.
3. Cook for about 5-7 minutes, or until the berries soften and release their juices, and the mixture thickens slightly.
4. Remove the saucepan from the heat and let the berry compote cool slightly.
5. Serve the low-potassium berry compote warm or chilled as a topping for yogurt, oatmeal, pancakes, or ice cream.

Nutritional Values (Approximate):

Calories: 40-50 kcal | Protein: 0.5-1 gram | Fat: 0 grams | Carbohydrates: 10-12 grams | Fiber: 2-3 grams | Sugars: 8-10 grams

Low-Potassium Fruit Salad:

Prep Time: 10 minutes
Chill Time: 30 minutes
Servings: 4

Ingredients:

- 2 cups mixed fresh fruits (such as diced apples, sliced bananas, grapes, kiwi, and melon)
- 1 tablespoon lemon juice
- 1 tablespoon honey or maple syrup (optional)
- Fresh mint leaves for garnish (optional)

Instructions:

1. In a large mixing bowl, combine mixed fresh fruits and lemon juice. Toss gently to coat the fruits with lemon juice to prevent browning.
2. If desired, drizzle honey or maple syrup over the fruit salad and toss again to combine.
3. Cover the fruit salad with plastic wrap and refrigerate for at least 30 minutes to allow the flavors to meld.
4. Before serving, garnish the low-potassium fruit salad with fresh mint leaves if desired.

Nutritional Values (Approximate):

Calories: 60-80 kcal | Protein: 0.5-1 gram | Fat: 0 grams | Carbohydrates: 15-20 grams | Fiber: 2-3 grams | Sugars: 10-15 grams

Tips for Enjoying Desserts in Moderation

1. **Portion Control:** Serve yourself a small portion of dessert rather than indulging in large servings. Use smaller plates or bowls to help control portion sizes.

2. **Savor Each Bite:** Take your time to fully enjoy each bite of dessert. Pay attention to the flavors, textures, and aromas. Eating slowly can help you feel more satisfied with less food.

3. **Choose Quality Over Quantity:** Opt for high-quality desserts made with wholesome ingredients whenever possible. Treat yourself to homemade desserts or those made with natural sweeteners and whole grains.

4. **Plan Ahead:** Incorporate desserts into your meal plan in moderation. If you know you'll be having dessert, adjust your meals accordingly to balance your calorie intake for the day.

5. **Mindful Eating:** Be mindful of your hunger and fullness cues. Stop eating when you feel satisfied rather than continuing to eat out of habit or temptation.

6. **Stay Hydrated:** Drink water or herbal tea before and after enjoying dessert. Sometimes thirst can be mistaken for hunger, leading to overeating.

7. **Share Desserts:** Split desserts with a friend or family member when dining out. Sharing allows you to enjoy a taste of something sweet without consuming a full portion.

8. **Practice Balance:** Balance indulgent desserts with healthier food choices throughout the day. Aim to include plenty of fruits, vegetables, whole grains, and lean proteins in your diet.

9. **Be Kind to Yourself:** Remember that it's okay to indulge in dessert occasionally. Avoid feelings of guilt or deprivation, and instead, focus on enjoying the experience.

10. **Listen to Your Body:** Pay attention to how your body feels after eating dessert. If certain desserts make you feel sluggish or uncomfortable, consider alternatives that better suit your body's needs.

Chapter 9: Beverages and Hydration

Beverages play a significant role in hydration and overall health. Here are some guidelines for maintaining hydration and making healthier beverage choices:

1. **Drink Plenty of Water:** Water is essential for hydration and overall health. Aim to drink at least 8 glasses of water per day, or more if you're physically active or in hot weather. Carry a reusable water bottle with you to stay hydrated throughout the day.

2. **Limit Sugary Drinks:** Sugary beverages like soda, fruit juices, sweetened teas, and sports drinks can contribute to weight gain and increase the risk of chronic diseases like diabetes and heart disease. Limit your intake of these drinks and opt for healthier alternatives instead.

3. **Choose Unsweetened Beverages:** Opt for unsweetened beverages whenever possible. Choose plain water, sparkling water, herbal teas, and unsweetened coffee or tea to reduce your intake of added sugars.

4. **Watch Your Alcohol Intake:** While moderate alcohol consumption may have some health benefits, excessive alcohol intake can lead to dehydration, liver damage, and other health problems. If you choose to drink alcohol, do so in moderation and be mindful of your intake.

5. **Be Cautious with Energy Drinks:** Energy drinks often contain high levels of caffeine and sugar, which can lead to dehydration and other health issues. Limit your intake of energy drinks, especially if you have underlying health conditions or are sensitive to caffeine.

6. **Incorporate Low-Calorie Options:** If you're looking to reduce your calorie intake, consider incorporating low-calorie beverages like flavored sparkling water, unsweetened almond milk, or coconut water into your diet.

7. **Read Labels:** Pay attention to the nutrition labels on beverage packaging to understand the ingredients and nutritional content. Look for drinks with minimal added sugars, artificial sweeteners, and other additives.

8. **Stay Hydrated During Exercise:** Drink water before, during, and after exercise to stay hydrated and replace lost fluids. Consider sports drinks if you're engaging in prolonged or intense physical activity to replenish electrolytes lost through sweat.

9. **Experiment with Infused Water:** Add natural flavor to your water by infusing it with fruits, vegetables, or herbs. Try combinations like cucumber and mint, lemon and ginger, or berries and basil for a refreshing and hydrating twist.

10. **Listen to Your Body:** Pay attention to your body's thirst cues and drink water whenever you feel thirsty. Additionally, monitor the color of your urine, aiming for pale yellow, which indicates proper hydration.

Importance of Hydration for Kidney Function

1. **Maintains Fluid Balance:** Adequate hydration helps maintain the balance of fluids and electrolytes in the body. Proper fluid balance is essential for kidney function as the kidneys regulate the concentration of electrolytes like sodium, potassium, and chloride in the blood.

2. **Supports Waste Removal:** The kidneys filter waste products and toxins from the blood to be excreted in the urine. Sufficient water intake ensures that the kidneys can effectively flush out waste products, toxins, and excess minerals from the body.

3. **Prevents Kidney Stones:** Dehydration can lead to the formation of kidney stones. When urine becomes concentrated due to insufficient fluid intake, minerals and salts can crystallize and form stones in the kidneys or urinary tract. Drinking enough water helps prevent the buildup of minerals and reduces the risk of kidney stone formation.

4. **Promotes Blood Pressure Regulation:** Adequate hydration helps regulate blood pressure, which is important for kidney health. The kidneys play a key role in blood pressure regulation by adjusting the volume of blood circulating in the body and releasing hormones that control blood vessel constriction and dilation. Dehydration can lead to increased blood pressure, which can strain the kidneys over time.

5. **Enhances Blood Flow to the Kidneys:** Proper hydration ensures adequate blood flow to the kidneys, which is necessary for their function. When the body is dehydrated, blood volume decreases, leading to reduced blood flow to the kidneys. This can impair kidney function and increase the risk of kidney damage.

6. **Supports Acid-Base Balance:** The kidneys help maintain the body's acid-base balance by excreting hydrogen ions and regulating bicarbonate levels in the blood. Adequate hydration is essential for this process to function optimally.

7. **Reduces the Risk of Kidney Disease:** Chronic dehydration can contribute to the development of kidney disease over time. By staying well-hydrated, you can help protect your kidneys from damage and reduce the risk of developing kidney-related conditions such as chronic kidney disease (CKD).

8. **Facilitates Medication Clearance:** Proper hydration ensures that medications and metabolic waste products are effectively cleared from the body through urine. Inadequate fluid intake can impair the kidneys' ability to filter and eliminate medications and toxins, potentially leading to medication toxicity or other adverse effects.

Kidney-Friendly Beverage Options

1. **Water:** Plain water is the best choice for kidney health. It helps maintain hydration, supports kidney function, and assists in flushing out waste products from the body. Aim to drink plenty of water throughout the day to stay hydrated.

2. **Herbal Teas:** Herbal teas made from kidney-friendly herbs like hibiscus, chamomile, ginger, and dandelion root can be soothing and hydrating. These teas are caffeine-free and may have additional health benefits such as reducing inflammation and supporting digestion.

3. **Fruit-Infused Water:** Add natural flavor to your water by infusing it with slices of fruits like lemon, lime, orange, cucumber, or berries. This adds a refreshing twist to plain water without the added sugars or artificial flavors found in many commercial beverages.

4. **Coconut Water:** Coconut water is a natural source of electrolytes like potassium and magnesium, which can help replenish lost fluids and electrolytes due to sweating or dehydration. It's lower in potassium compared to sports drinks and is a good option for occasional hydration.

5. **Diluted Fruit Juices:** While fruit juices can be high in natural sugars and potassium, diluting them with water can help reduce their sugar and potassium content while still providing flavor. Opt for juices that are lower in potassium, such as apple or cranberry juice, and dilute them with water to lower their potassium concentration.

6. **Low-Sodium Vegetable Juice:** Vegetable juices can be a nutritious option for kidney health, especially when they are low in sodium. Look for vegetable juices that are low in sodium or make your own at home using fresh vegetables like carrots, celery, spinach, and kale.

7. **Almond Milk or Rice Milk:** For those who need to limit dairy intake due to kidney-related issues, almond milk or rice milk can be suitable alternatives. Choose unsweetened varieties to avoid added sugars and watch out for phosphorus additives in fortified versions.

8. **Sparkling Water:** Sparkling water or seltzer can be a refreshing alternative to plain water for those who prefer a bit of fizz. Look for unsweetened varieties without added flavors or sugars.

9. **Homemade Smoothies:** Make your own kidney-friendly smoothies using ingredients like low-potassium fruits (e.g., berries, apples), leafy greens, almond milk, and a small amount of protein powder or nut butter for added nutrition. Avoid adding high-potassium ingredients like bananas or oranges.

10. **Decaffeinated Coffee and Tea:** If you enjoy coffee or tea, opt for decaffeinated versions, as caffeine can have diuretic effects and may increase blood pressure. Decaffeinated coffee and tea can still provide the comforting taste without the stimulating effects of caffeine.

Strategies for Monitoring Fluid Intake

1. **Keep a Fluid Intake Diary:** Record all fluids consumed throughout the day in a diary or journal. Include details such as the type of beverage, quantity consumed, and the time of consumption. This can help you track your fluid intake accurately and identify any patterns or trends over time.

2. **Set Daily Fluid Goals:** Work with your healthcare provider or dietitian to determine an appropriate daily fluid intake goal based on your individual needs, medical condition, and level of physical activity. Use this goal as a benchmark to guide your fluid intake and ensure you're meeting your hydration needs.

3. **Measure Fluids:** Use measuring cups, glasses with marked measurements, or water bottles with predefined volumes to measure the quantity of fluids consumed accurately. This can help you control portion sizes and avoid overconsumption.

4. **Monitor Urine Output:** Pay attention to the frequency and volume of urination as a gauge of your hydration status. Adequate fluid intake typically results in pale yellow urine, while dark yellow or concentrated urine may indicate dehydration. However, certain medications or medical conditions can affect urine color, so it's essential to consult with a healthcare professional for personalized guidance.

5. **Use Technology:** Consider using smartphone apps or digital tools designed to track fluid intake. These apps allow you to log your beverages easily, set reminders for drinking fluids throughout the day, and generate reports to monitor your progress over time.

6. **Be Mindful of Hidden Fluids:** Be aware of hidden sources of fluids in foods such as soups, fruits, vegetables, and dairy products. While these foods contribute to overall hydration, it's essential to account for their fluid content when monitoring your total fluid intake.

7. **Limit Fluids During Meals:** Avoid consuming large volumes of fluids with meals, as this can interfere with digestion and increase the risk of fluid overload. Instead, drink small amounts of fluids between meals to maintain hydration without overwhelming your kidneys.

8. **Monitor Weight Changes:** Regularly weigh yourself at the same time each day, preferably in the morning before eating or drinking. Sudden weight changes can indicate

shifts in fluid balance, such as fluid retention or dehydration. Consult with your healthcare provider if you notice significant fluctuations in weight.

9. **Seek Professional Guidance:** Work closely with your healthcare team, including your nephrologist, dietitian, or primary care provider, to develop a personalized fluid management plan tailored to your specific needs and medical condition. They can provide expert advice, monitor your progress, and make adjustments as needed.

Chapter 10: Managing Special Dietary Needs

Managing special dietary needs, especially in the context of kidney disease or other kidney-related conditions, requires careful planning and adherence to specific guidelines to support overall health and well-being. Here are some strategies for effectively managing special dietary needs:

1. **Consult with a Registered Dietitian:** A registered dietitian specializing in kidney health can provide personalized dietary recommendations tailored to your individual needs, medical history, and dietary preferences. They can help you understand your dietary restrictions, plan balanced meals, and make informed food choices to support kidney function.

2. **Understand Dietary Restrictions:** Educate yourself about specific dietary restrictions associated with your condition, such as limiting sodium, potassium, phosphorus, and protein intake. Understanding the rationale behind these restrictions can help you make informed decisions about food selection and meal preparation.

3. **Monitor Nutrient Intake:** Keep track of your daily nutrient intake, including sodium, potassium, phosphorus, protein, and fluid intake. Use food labels, nutrition databases, or smartphone apps to calculate nutrient content and ensure compliance with dietary recommendations.

4. **Choose Kidney-Friendly Foods:** Focus on incorporating kidney-friendly foods into your diet, such as fresh fruits and vegetables (with limited potassium), lean proteins, whole grains, and healthy fats. Avoid processed and packaged foods high in sodium, phosphorus additives, and hidden sugars.

5. **Practice Portion Control:** Pay attention to portion sizes to prevent overconsumption of nutrients that may be harmful to kidney health, such as protein, phosphorus, and potassium. Use measuring cups, food scales, or visual cues to control portion sizes and avoid excess calorie intake.

6. **Limit Phosphorus-Containing Foods:** Reduce consumption of foods high in phosphorus, such as dairy products, nuts, seeds, whole grains, and processed foods with phosphate additives. Choose lower-phosphorus alternatives and consider using phosphorus binders as prescribed by your healthcare provider.

7. **Monitor Fluid Intake:** Maintain adequate hydration by monitoring fluid intake and adhering to recommended fluid restrictions if necessary. Limit fluids containing high levels of sodium, potassium, or phosphorus, and choose hydrating beverages like water, herbal teas, and diluted fruit juices.

8. **Modify Cooking Techniques:** Adopt cooking methods that minimize the use of added fats, oils, and salt while preserving the natural flavors of foods. Opt for baking, grilling, steaming, or sautéing with minimal oil instead of frying or deep-frying. Experiment with herbs, spices, and citrus juices to enhance flavor without adding extra sodium.

9. **Read Food Labels:** Become proficient at reading food labels to identify hidden sources of sodium, potassium, and phosphorus in packaged foods. Look for low-sodium, low-potassium, and low-phosphorus alternatives, and avoid products with phosphorus additives like sodium phosphate or potassium phosphate.

10. **Stay Informed and Updated:** Keep abreast of the latest research, guidelines, and recommendations related to your dietary needs and kidney health. Attend educational sessions, join support groups, and consult reliable sources of information to stay informed and empowered in managing your special dietary needs.

Diabetes and Kidney Disease: Dietary Considerations

When managing both diabetes and kidney disease, dietary considerations play a critical role in maintaining optimal health and preventing complications.

1. **Control Blood Sugar Levels:** Aim to stabilize blood sugar levels through consistent carbohydrate intake spread throughout the day. Choose complex carbohydrates with a low glycemic index to minimize spikes in blood sugar levels. Monitor carbohydrate intake and adjust insulin or medication doses as needed.

2. **Manage Protein Intake:** Limit protein intake to reduce the workload on the kidneys and prevent further kidney damage. Choose high-quality protein sources such as lean meats, poultry, fish, eggs, and plant-based proteins like legumes, tofu, and tempeh. Monitor portion sizes and consult with a dietitian to determine the appropriate amount of protein for your individual needs.

3. **Limit Sodium Intake:** Reduce sodium intake to help control blood pressure and manage fluid retention, which are common concerns in both diabetes and kidney disease. Avoid processed and packaged foods high in sodium and limit the use of salt in cooking. Choose fresh, whole foods and use herbs, spices, and lemon juice to flavor dishes instead of salt.

4. **Control Phosphorus and Potassium:** Monitor phosphorus and potassium intake, as imbalances can occur in kidney disease and affect bone health and heart function. Limit high-phosphorus foods such as dairy products, nuts, seeds, and processed foods. Choose lower-potassium fruits and vegetables and leach potassium from vegetables by soaking them in water before cooking.

5. **Emphasize Plant-Based Foods:** Incorporate a variety of fruits, vegetables, whole grains, and legumes into your diet to provide essential nutrients, fiber, and antioxidants. Plant-based foods are generally lower in saturated fat and cholesterol, which can benefit heart health and overall well-being.

6. **Stay Hydrated:** Drink plenty of water to maintain hydration and support kidney function. Aim for at least 8-10 cups of fluid per day, adjusting intake based on individual needs and fluid restrictions. Choose water, herbal teas, and other low-calorie, low-sugar beverages over sugary drinks and sodas.

7. **Monitor Blood Pressure:** Keep blood pressure under control by following a heart-healthy diet rich in fruits, vegetables, whole grains, lean proteins, and healthy fats. Limit alcohol intake, manage stress, and engage in regular physical activity to help lower blood pressure and reduce the risk of cardiovascular complications.

8. **Monitor Blood Lipids:** Pay attention to blood lipid levels (cholesterol and triglycerides) and follow a diet low in saturated and trans fats to help manage lipid levels

and reduce the risk of cardiovascular disease. Choose healthy fats from sources like nuts, seeds, avocados, and olive oil in moderation.

9. **Individualize Your Diet:** Work closely with a registered dietitian who specializes in diabetes and kidney disease to develop a personalized meal plan tailored to your specific needs, preferences, and medical condition. Regular monitoring and adjustments to your diet may be necessary to achieve optimal blood sugar control, kidney function, and overall health.

10. **Educate Yourself:** Take an active role in learning about nutrition, diabetes management, and kidney disease to make informed decisions about your diet and lifestyle. Stay up-to-date on the latest research, guidelines, and recommendations from reputable sources, and ask questions to your healthcare team when in doubt.

Heart Health and Kidney Disease: Incorporating Heart-Healthy Eating

1. **Focus on Plant-Based Foods:** Emphasize fruits, vegetables, whole grains, legumes, nuts, and seeds in your diet. These foods are rich in fiber, vitamins, minerals, and antioxidants, which support heart health and overall well-being. Aim to fill half your plate with colorful plant-based foods at each meal.

2. **Choose Lean Proteins:** Opt for lean protein sources such as skinless poultry, fish, tofu, tempeh, legumes, and low-fat dairy products. Limit red meat and processed meats, as they are high in saturated fat and sodium, which can increase the risk of heart disease and exacerbate kidney issues.

3. **Limit Saturated and Trans Fats:** Reduce intake of saturated and trans fats, which can raise cholesterol levels and contribute to heart disease. Choose heart-healthy fats from sources like olive oil, avocados, nuts, and seeds. Limit fried foods, baked goods, processed snacks, and fatty cuts of meat.

4. **Monitor Sodium Intake:** Limit sodium intake to help control blood pressure and reduce fluid retention. Choose fresh or minimally processed foods and season meals with herbs, spices, lemon juice, or vinegar instead of salt. Aim for less than 2,300 milligrams of sodium per day, or even lower if advised by your healthcare provider.

5. **Control Phosphorus and Potassium:** Keep phosphorus and potassium levels in check by choosing low-phosphorus and low-potassium foods. Limit high-phosphorus foods such as dairy products, nuts, seeds, and processed foods with phosphate additives. Choose lower-potassium fruits and vegetables and leach potassium from vegetables before cooking.

6. **Monitor Fluid Intake:** Stay hydrated by drinking plenty of water throughout the day, but be mindful of fluid restrictions if advised by your healthcare provider. Limit fluid intake from sugary beverages, alcohol, and caffeinated drinks, as they can contribute to dehydration and negatively impact heart and kidney health.

7. **Control Blood Sugar Levels:** Manage blood sugar levels through consistent carbohydrate intake and portion control. Choose complex carbohydrates with a low glycemic index to prevent spikes in blood sugar levels. Monitor carbohydrate intake and adjust insulin or medication doses as needed to maintain stable blood sugar levels.

8. **Maintain a Healthy Weight:** Strive to achieve and maintain a healthy weight through a balanced diet and regular physical activity. Excess weight can strain the heart and kidneys, leading to complications such as high blood pressure and diabetes. Aim for gradual weight loss if overweight or obese, under the guidance of a healthcare professional.

9. **Limit Alcohol Consumption:** Drink alcohol in moderation, if at all, as excessive alcohol consumption can raise blood pressure and contribute to heart disease and kidney

damage. Limit intake to one drink per day for women and up to two drinks per day for men, following recommended guidelines.

10. **Stay Active:** Engage in regular physical activity to promote heart health, maintain muscle strength, and improve overall well-being. Aim for at least 150 minutes of moderate-intensity exercise per week, such as brisk walking, cycling, swimming, or dancing. Consult with your healthcare provider before starting any new exercise program.

Gluten-Free and Dairy-Free Options for Dietary Restrictions

Gluten-Free Options:

1. **Whole Grains:** Incorporate gluten-free grains such as quinoa, brown rice, millet, amaranth, buckwheat, and gluten-free oats into your diet. These grains provide fiber, vitamins, and minerals while being free from gluten.

2. **Vegetables and Fruits:** Load up on a variety of fresh fruits and vegetables, which are naturally gluten-free and packed with essential nutrients, antioxidants, and fiber.

3. **Lean Proteins:** Choose lean protein sources such as poultry, fish, seafood, eggs, legumes, tofu, tempeh, and nuts, which are naturally gluten-free and provide essential amino acids.

4. **Dairy Alternatives:** Opt for dairy-free milk alternatives like almond milk, coconut milk, soy milk, rice milk, or oat milk. These alternatives are fortified with calcium and vitamin D to support bone health.

5. **Healthy Fats:** Include sources of healthy fats such as avocados, olive oil, coconut oil, nuts, and seeds in your diet to provide essential fatty acids and promote heart health.

6. **Gluten-Free Grains:** Experiment with gluten-free grains and flours in baking and cooking, including almond flour, coconut flour, chickpea flour, tapioca flour, and sorghum flour.

7. **Gluten-Free Snacks:** Choose gluten-free snacks such as popcorn, rice cakes, gluten-free crackers, nuts, seeds, and fruit to satisfy cravings between meals.

Dairy-Free Options:

1. **Plant-Based Milks:** Use plant-based milk alternatives such as almond milk, coconut milk, soy milk, rice milk, or oat milk in place of cow's milk in recipes, cereals, smoothies, and beverages.

2. **Non-Dairy Yogurts:** Enjoy non-dairy yogurt made from coconut milk, almond milk, soy milk, or cashew milk, which provides probiotics and nutrients similar to dairy yogurt.

3. **Cheese Alternatives:** Explore dairy-free cheese alternatives made from nuts (such as almond or cashew cheese), soy, or coconut, which can be used in recipes or as toppings.

4. **Cooking Substitutes:** Use dairy-free alternatives such as coconut oil, olive oil, or dairy-free margarine in cooking and baking instead of butter or ghee.

5. **Plant-Based Proteins:** Incorporate plant-based protein sources such as beans, lentils, tofu, tempeh, edamame, quinoa, and nuts to meet your protein needs without relying on dairy products.

6. **Read Labels:** When purchasing packaged or processed foods, always read labels carefully to check for hidden sources of gluten or dairy, as these ingredients may be present in unexpected products.

7. **Homemade Meals:** Prepare homemade meals using fresh, whole ingredients to have better control over the ingredients and ensure your meals are gluten-free and dairy-free.

Strategies for Dining Out and Social Gatherings

Dining Out:

1. **Research Restaurants:** Before going out, research restaurants in your area that offer gluten-free and dairy-free options. Many restaurants now provide special menus or indicate allergen information on their websites.

2. **Communicate with Staff:** Inform your server about your dietary restrictions when you arrive at the restaurant. Ask questions about menu items, ingredients, and how dishes are prepared to ensure they meet your needs.

3. **Ask for Modifications:** Don't hesitate to ask for modifications to menu items to make them gluten-free or dairy-free. Many restaurants are willing to accommodate dietary restrictions and can adjust dishes accordingly.

4. **Focus on Naturally Gluten-Free and Dairy-Free Foods:** Choose dishes that are naturally gluten-free and dairy-free, such as grilled meats, fish, salads, and vegetable-based dishes. Be cautious of sauces, dressings, and marinades that may contain gluten or dairy.

5. **Avoid Cross-Contamination:** Ask about cross-contamination risks, especially if you have celiac disease or severe food allergies. Request that utensils, cookware, and preparation surfaces be thoroughly cleaned to prevent cross-contact with gluten or dairy.

6. **Bring Your Own Condiments:** Consider bringing your own gluten-free soy sauce, dairy-free salad dressings, or condiments to add flavor to your meal if the restaurant doesn't offer suitable options.

Social Gatherings:

1. **Communicate in Advance:** If you're attending a social gathering or party, communicate your dietary restrictions to the host in advance. Offer to bring a dish or snacks that you can enjoy and share with others.

2. **Bring Your Own Food:** To ensure you have safe options to eat, bring your own gluten-free and dairy-free dishes or snacks to social events. This way, you'll have something you can enjoy without worrying about ingredients.

3. **Focus on Safe Options:** Scan the buffet or food spread for naturally gluten-free and dairy-free options, such as fresh fruits, vegetables, nuts, and plain meats. Be cautious of dishes that may contain hidden gluten or dairy ingredients.

4. **Be Prepared to Explain:** Be prepared to explain your dietary restrictions to others at the gathering who may not be familiar with gluten-free or dairy-free diets. Politely educate them about your needs and why certain foods are off-limits.

5. **Enjoy the Company:** While food is often a central focus of social gatherings, remember that the primary purpose is to enjoy the company of friends and family. Focus on the social aspect of the event rather than solely on the food.

6. **Plan Ahead:** If you're unsure whether there will be suitable options available, eat a snack before the event to prevent hunger and make it easier to navigate the food choices available.

Chapter 11: Lifestyle Tips for Kidney Health

Maintaining a healthy lifestyle is crucial for kidney health, especially for individuals with kidney disease or those at risk of developing it. Here are some lifestyle tips to promote kidney health:

1. **Stay Hydrated:** Drink plenty of water throughout the day to keep your kidneys functioning optimally. Adequate hydration helps flush toxins and waste products from the body, reducing the risk of kidney stones and urinary tract infections.

2. **Follow a Balanced Diet:** Adopt a diet rich in fruits, vegetables, whole grains, lean proteins, and healthy fats. Limit intake of processed foods, saturated fats, refined sugars, and excessive salt, which can strain the kidneys and contribute to high blood pressure and kidney damage.

3. **Monitor Blood Pressure:** Keep your blood pressure in check by maintaining a healthy weight, limiting sodium intake, exercising regularly, and managing stress. High blood pressure can damage the kidneys over time, leading to kidney disease.

4. **Control Blood Sugar:** If you have diabetes, monitor your blood sugar levels closely and follow your healthcare provider's recommendations for managing your condition. Elevated blood sugar levels can damage the kidneys and increase the risk of diabetic nephropathy.

5. **Maintain a Healthy Weight:** Aim for a healthy weight through a balanced diet and regular exercise. Obesity is a risk factor for kidney disease and can contribute to high blood pressure, diabetes, and other conditions that affect kidney health.

6. **Exercise Regularly:** Engage in regular physical activity to support overall health and well-being. Exercise helps control weight, lower blood pressure, improve circulation, and reduce the risk of chronic diseases that can impact kidney function.

7. **Quit Smoking:** If you smoke, take steps to quit smoking as soon as possible. Smoking damages blood vessels and impairs kidney function, increasing the risk of kidney disease and other health problems.

8. **Limit Alcohol Consumption:** Drink alcohol in moderation, as excessive alcohol consumption can affect kidney function and increase the risk of liver disease and other health issues.

9. **Manage Stress:** Find healthy ways to manage stress, such as practicing relaxation techniques, mindfulness, meditation, or engaging in hobbies and activities you enjoy. Chronic stress can contribute to high blood pressure and negatively impact kidney health.

10. **Get Regular Check-ups:** Schedule regular check-ups with your healthcare provider to monitor your kidney function and overall health. Early detection and management of kidney disease and related conditions can help prevent complications and preserve kidney function.

Exercise and Physical Activity Recommendations

1. **Aerobic Exercise:** Engage in regular aerobic exercise, such as brisk walking, jogging, cycling, swimming, or dancing, for at least 150 minutes per week. Aerobic exercise improves cardiovascular health, helps control weight, and promotes overall fitness.

2. **Strength Training:** Incorporate strength training exercises, such as weightlifting, bodyweight exercises, or resistance band workouts, at least two days per week. Strength training helps build muscle mass, improve bone density, and enhance metabolism.

3. **Flexibility and Stretching:** Perform flexibility and stretching exercises to improve range of motion, reduce stiffness, and prevent injury. Include stretches for major muscle groups, focusing on areas prone to tightness, such as the hips, hamstrings, and shoulders.

4. **Balance and Stability Training:** Include balance and stability exercises, such as yoga, tai chi, or Pilates, to enhance coordination, proprioception, and posture. Balance training reduces the risk of falls and improves overall functional fitness.

5. **Gradual Progression:** Start slowly and gradually increase the intensity, duration, and frequency of your workouts over time. Listen to your body and avoid overexertion, especially if you're new to exercise or have existing health conditions.

6. **Stay Active Throughout the Day:** Incorporate physical activity into your daily routine by taking the stairs instead of the elevator, walking or cycling for short trips, and finding opportunities to move throughout the day, such as gardening or household chores.

7. **Hydration:** Stay hydrated before, during, and after exercise by drinking water or electrolyte-replenishing beverages. Proper hydration is essential for optimal kidney function and helps regulate body temperature during physical activity.

8. **Warm-up and Cool-down:** Always warm up before exercise with dynamic stretches or light aerobic activity to prepare your muscles and joints for movement. After your workout, cool down with static stretches to promote muscle recovery and flexibility.

9. **Listen to Your Body:** Pay attention to how your body responds to exercise and adjust your routine as needed. If you experience pain, discomfort, or unusual symptoms during or after exercise, consult with a healthcare professional.

10. **Consult with Your Healthcare Provider:** Before starting a new exercise program, especially if you have underlying health conditions or concerns about kidney health, consult with your healthcare provider or a qualified exercise specialist for personalized recommendations and guidance.

Stress Management Techniques for Overall Wellness

1. **Mindfulness Meditation:** Practice mindfulness meditation to cultivate present-moment awareness and reduce stress. Focus on your breath, bodily sensations, or a specific object without judgment. Regular meditation can help calm the mind and enhance relaxation.

2. **Deep Breathing Exercises:** Engage in deep breathing exercises to activate the body's relaxation response and reduce stress. Practice diaphragmatic breathing by inhaling deeply through your nose, expanding your abdomen, and exhaling slowly through your mouth.

3. **Progressive Muscle Relaxation (PMR):** Practice PMR to systematically tense and relax different muscle groups in your body. Start with your toes and work your way up to your head, tensing each muscle group for a few seconds before releasing the tension.

4. **Yoga and Tai Chi:** Participate in yoga or tai chi classes to promote relaxation, flexibility, and mindfulness. These mind-body practices combine gentle movements with breath awareness and meditation to reduce stress and improve overall well-being.

5. **Physical Activity:** Engage in regular physical activity to reduce stress hormones and boost mood-enhancing endorphins. Choose activities you enjoy, such as walking, jogging, cycling, or dancing, and aim for at least 30 minutes of exercise most days of the week.

6. **Healthy Lifestyle Habits:** Adopt healthy lifestyle habits, such as eating a balanced diet, getting adequate sleep, and avoiding excessive alcohol and caffeine consumption. These lifestyle factors can support resilience to stress and promote overall wellness.

7. **Social Support:** Seek support from friends, family members, or support groups during times of stress. Sharing your feelings and experiences with others can provide emotional validation and perspective, reducing feelings of isolation and anxiety.

8. **Time Management:** Practice effective time management techniques to prioritize tasks, set realistic goals, and delegate responsibilities. Breaking tasks into smaller, manageable steps can reduce feelings of overwhelm and improve productivity.

9. **Relaxation Techniques:** Explore different relaxation techniques, such as guided imagery, aromatherapy, or listening to soothing music. Find activities that help you unwind and promote relaxation, whether it's taking a warm bath, enjoying nature, or practicing a hobby.

10. **Seek Professional Help:** If stress becomes overwhelming or interferes with your daily functioning, consider seeking support from a mental health professional. Therapy, counseling, or stress management programs can provide tools and strategies to cope with stress more effectively.

Importance of Regular Medical Monitoring and Follow-Up Care

1. **Early Detection of Kidney Disease:** Regular monitoring allows healthcare providers to detect kidney disease in its early stages when treatment and intervention can be most effective. Early detection enables timely management of risk factors and implementation of strategies to slow the progression of kidney disease.

2. **Assessment of Kidney Function:** Routine tests, such as blood and urine tests, help assess kidney function by measuring markers like creatinine, blood urea nitrogen (BUN), and glomerular filtration rate (GFR). Monitoring changes in these markers over time provides valuable insights into kidney health and allows for appropriate interventions as needed.

3. **Management of Chronic Conditions:** Many chronic conditions, such as diabetes, hypertension, and autoimmune disorders, can impact kidney function. Regular medical monitoring allows healthcare providers to manage these underlying conditions effectively, reducing the risk of kidney complications and disease progression.

4. **Medication Management:** Patients with kidney disease often require medications to manage symptoms, control blood pressure, and prevent complications. Regular follow-up appointments allow healthcare providers to monitor medication effectiveness, adjust dosages as needed, and minimize adverse effects.

5. **Prevention of Complications:** Kidney disease can lead to various complications, including cardiovascular disease, anemia, bone disorders, and electrolyte imbalances. Regular medical monitoring helps identify and address these complications early, preventing further deterioration of kidney function and improving overall health outcomes.

6. **Nutritional Assessment and Counseling:** Nutrition plays a crucial role in managing kidney disease and supporting overall health. Regular follow-up care may include nutritional assessment and counseling to optimize dietary choices, manage electrolyte imbalances, and prevent malnutrition.

7. **Coordination of Care:** Regular follow-up appointments facilitate coordination of care among healthcare providers, including nephrologists, primary care physicians, dietitians, and other specialists. This interdisciplinary approach ensures comprehensive management of kidney disease and associated comorbidities.

8. **Patient Education and Empowerment:** Regular medical monitoring provides opportunities for patient education and empowerment. Healthcare providers can educate patients about kidney disease, treatment options, lifestyle modifications, self-care strategies, and resources for support, empowering patients to actively participate in their care and make informed decisions.

9. **Monitoring Treatment Response:** For patients receiving treatment for kidney disease, such as dialysis or kidney transplantation, regular follow-up appointments allow healthcare providers to monitor treatment response, address complications, and optimize outcomes.

10. **Quality of Life Improvement:** By closely monitoring kidney health and providing timely interventions, regular medical monitoring and follow-up care can improve the quality of life for patients with kidney disease, enabling them to live fuller, healthier lives.

Encouragement and Support for Continued Success

As you embark on your journey to manage kidney disease through diet and lifestyle changes, it's essential to remember that every step you take towards better health is a significant achievement. Here are some words of encouragement and support to keep you motivated along the way:

1. **You're Not Alone:** Remember that you are not alone in this journey. There is a supportive community of healthcare professionals, family, friends, and fellow individuals managing kidney disease who are here to offer guidance, encouragement, and understanding.

2. **Celebrate Progress:** Celebrate every small victory and progress you make towards improving your kidney health. Whether it's sticking to your dietary plan, incorporating more physical activity into your routine, or attending regular medical appointments, each step forward is worth acknowledging and celebrating.

3. **Stay Positive:** Maintain a positive outlook and focus on what you can control. While managing kidney disease may present challenges, maintaining a positive attitude can help you navigate through them with resilience and determination.

4. **Set Realistic Goals:** Set realistic and achievable goals for yourself, whether it's reaching a certain milestone in your dietary plan, increasing your exercise regimen gradually, or improving your overall well-being. Break down larger goals into smaller, manageable steps to make progress more attainable.

5. **Practice Self-Compassion:** Be kind to yourself and practice self-compassion throughout your journey. Understand that setbacks may occur, but they are opportunities for growth and learning. Treat yourself with the same care and compassion you would offer to a loved one facing similar challenges.

6. **Seek Support:** Don't hesitate to reach out for support when needed. Lean on your support network, including healthcare providers, family, friends, and support groups, for encouragement, advice, and understanding. Sharing your experiences and challenges with others can provide valuable insights and solidarity.

7. **Stay Informed:** Stay informed about the latest developments in kidney health, dietary recommendations, and treatment options. Knowledge empowers you to make informed decisions about your health and advocate for yourself effectively.

8. **Practice Self-Care:** Prioritize self-care activities that promote your physical, emotional, and mental well-being. Whether it's engaging in hobbies you enjoy, practicing relaxation

techniques, or spending quality time with loved ones, make time for activities that rejuvenate and nourish your soul.

9. **Stay Persistent:** Remember that managing kidney disease is a journey that requires ongoing effort and persistence. Stay committed to your health goals, even when faced with challenges or setbacks, and trust in your ability to overcome obstacles along the way.

10. **Believe in Yourself:** Believe in your strength, resilience, and ability to navigate through life's challenges, including managing kidney disease. You have the power within you to take control of your health, make positive changes, and lead a fulfilling life.

Conversion Charts for Nutritional Values

In the appendix of your "Kidney Disease Diet Cookbook for Men," you can include conversion charts for nutritional values to assist readers in understanding and utilizing the nutritional information provided in the recipes. Here's a suggested format for the conversion charts:

1. **Calories Conversion Chart:**
   - Provide a table that converts kilocalories (kcal) to calories (cal) for common serving sizes, such as 100 grams or 1 cup, to help readers accurately assess the calorie content of foods.

2. **Protein Conversion Chart:**
   - Offer a chart that converts grams of protein to other common units of measurement, such as ounces or milligrams, to help readers track their protein intake more effectively.

3. **Fat Conversion Chart:**
   - Provide a conversion table that converts grams of fat to other units, such as teaspoons or tablespoons, to assist readers in monitoring their fat consumption and portion sizes.

4. **Carbohydrates Conversion Chart:**
   - Include a chart that converts grams of carbohydrates to different units, such as grams, ounces, or servings, to help readers manage their carbohydrate intake and portion control.

5. **Fiber Conversion Chart:**
   - Offer a conversion table that converts grams of dietary fiber to other units, such as grams, ounces, or servings, to assist readers in meeting their fiber goals for improved digestive health.

6. **Sugars Conversion Chart:**
   - Provide a chart that converts grams of sugars to teaspoons or other units commonly used to measure sugar content, helping readers limit their sugar intake and make informed dietary choices.

7. **Sodium Conversion Chart:**
   - Include a conversion table that converts milligrams of sodium to other units, such as teaspoons of salt or grams of sodium chloride, to help readers reduce their sodium intake and monitor their salt consumption.

8. **Potassium Conversion Chart:**
   - Offer a chart that converts milligrams of potassium to other units, such as milliequivalents (mEq) or servings of potassium-rich foods, to assist readers in managing their potassium intake and avoiding hyperkalemia.

9. **Phosphorus Conversion Chart:**
   - Provide a conversion table that converts milligrams of phosphorus to other units, such as millimoles (mmol) or servings of phosphorus-containing foods, to help readers limit their phosphorus intake and maintain kidney health.

Sample Grocery Lists

1. **Basic Kidney-Friendly Grocery List:**
   - Include essential pantry staples and fresh produce items commonly used in kidney-friendly recipes, such as:
     - Whole grains: Brown rice, quinoa, whole wheat pasta
     - Lean proteins: Skinless chicken breast, turkey breast, fish (e.g., salmon, trout)
     - Low-fat dairy or dairy alternatives: Greek yogurt, almond milk, tofu
     - Fresh fruits and vegetables: Berries, apples, spinach, bell peppers, broccoli
     - Canned or dried beans: Kidney beans, black beans, lentils
     - Nuts and seeds: Almonds, walnuts, chia seeds
     - Cooking oils: Olive oil, avocado oil
     - Herbs and spices: Garlic, ginger, turmeric, parsley

2. **Weekly Meal Plan Grocery List:**
   - Provide a sample grocery list tailored to a week's worth of kidney-friendly meals, including ingredients for breakfast, lunch, dinner, and snacks. Organize the list by food categories or meals to make shopping more convenient for readers.

3. **Specialty Ingredients Grocery List:**
   - Offer a list of specialty ingredients or items that may not be commonly found in readers' pantries but are useful for preparing specific kidney-friendly dishes. This may include items like low-sodium broths, specialty flours, or alternative sweeteners.

4. **Seasonal Produce Shopping Guide:**
   - Create a guide that highlights seasonal fruits and vegetables suitable for kidney-friendly diets, along with tips for selecting, storing, and preparing these items. This can help readers make the most of seasonal produce and incorporate variety into their meals.

5. **Low-Sodium and Low-Phosphorus Product Recommendations:**
   - Recommend specific brands or products that are low in sodium and phosphorus, such as low-sodium canned goods, phosphorus-free snacks, and kidney-friendly condiments. Include tips for reading food labels and choosing healthier options.

www.ingramcontent.com/pod-product-compliance
Lightning Source LLC
Chambersburg PA
CBHW062110220526
45471CB00010B/3682